"Finally! A practical, refres[...] children of seniors."

— PAUL IARROBINO, Gatekeeper Coordinator,
Multnomah County Aging and Disabilities Services

"What a breath of fresh air for someone with an aging parent! Suzanne Roberts has artfully developed a straightforward, yet sensitive and meaningful resource for children of the elderly. Readers will quickly gain insightful knowledge and understanding on how to embrace the responsibilities and challenges of elder care. This book provides real peace of mind in the form of noteworthy advice and recommendations."

— PAUL HOGAN, President, Home Instead Senior Care

"*Coping in New Territory* is a must read for adult children of aging parents. Not only timely, it helps clarify roles and responsibilities, and suggests practical, loving, yet no-nonsense solutions to often very difficult situations. This handbook helps fill a major gap in understanding aging care and family relationships."

— JANET A. BAKER-KAHN,
MA, MFT Geriatric Mental Health Specialist

"This is an extremely valuable and useful book on how to successfully handle the many challenges of [caring for] aging parents. Suzanne Roberts shows great depth of experience with her practical, real-life suggestions on how to handle living arrangements, health care, and difficult emotional issues between parents and their adult children. Her book is like having a wise supportive, personal coach at your side. I'm especially impressed with her understanding of how old feelings stirred up by the new parent-child relationship can uncover hidden issues and lead to personal growth not possible in any other circumstance."

— AL SIEBERT, PHD.,
Author of *The Survivor Personality*

"What a wise and wonderful little book. And the binding is great. I know because my dog eared copy was read, consulted, underlined, and copied for the three months it took to convince, sort, pack, and move my 88 year old mother out of her own home. I know my guilt, anxiety, sleepless nights, and tears shed would have been far greater without this sturdy little book. Thank you."

— BARBARA LEAR
Literary Consultant, Book Strategies

COPING IN NEW TERRITORY

The Handbook for
Children of Aging Parents

SUZANNE ROBERTS

COPING IN NEW TERRITORY

The Handbook for
Children of Aging Parents

CHELTENHAM PRESS
Portland, Oregon

To my parents,
Fred and Barbara Ryan,
my greatest teachers
in sickness and in health

CONTENTS

ACKNOWLEDGMENTS

Hundreds of people influenced this book. It would be impossible to name them all, even if I knew their names. I attended scores of support groups and always came away with the germ of an idea, or a story I could tell in words that protected the people who so willingly shared. To all of you, thank you. A special thank you to Dr. Lynda Falkenstein, without her guidance on every aspect of this book, the book would never have been completed.

My gratitude to Nancy Osa, my editor, who made my words make sense to the reader, and to Claudine and Company who designed the beautiful cover and book interior. Thanks to Anna Browne for support and encouragement in the early stages of the writing. Hugs and thanks to Vivian Greenberg, who is a real author, and who helped me believe I was one, too. Thanks to Dr. Jeanne Jackson, who so lovingly helped my mother and by doing so was my teacher. I wanted the cover of the third edition to be more than a photograph of loving hands. I wanted the hands to be attached to people I cared about. One of my warmest memories will be the afternoon with photographer Leo Arfer; my darling 103 year old client Patricia Behrman and her niece Bonnie Vawter will always be one of my warmest memories. My thanks to these ladies for the laughter and love that was captured by Leo's camera. Thanks, finally, to my darling husband, Bud, who supported and encouraged me, gave me ideas when my mind was blank, fixed his own dinner when I was too busy to play wife, and demonstrated over and over how lucky I am to have found him.

FOREWORD

How did I go from being a fifty-six-year-old woman with grown children and four grandchildren to being an "adult child?" When my parents became ill, everything changed. I could no longer make travel reservations without buying cancellation insurance. My husband and I couldn't drop everything and go to the beach on the spur of the moment—not without notifying a substantial number of people how to reach us if we were needed. With the birth of my first child, I expected a loss of freedom. I didn't resent it. It was part of the responsibility of being a parent. As a woman in midlife, I deeply resented these new restrictions.

I had just married the man of my dreams. We were beginning our life together, and suddenly all my plans had to be put on hold. How was I going to solve this problem? I couldn't change the timing. I couldn't change the dementia that followed my mother's heart attack, or change the course of my father's lung cancer. I was a newlywed, not a caregiver! I had to find a way to be both.

So I asked myself, how do I lovingly care for my parents and have my own life? This book documents the answers I found over the next six years. Not everything written here will work in every situation, but most of the coping skills I present will work most of the time. Why? Because these skills come from love and caring. Not just love and caring for my parents, but love of my own life as well.

Since completing the first edition of *Coping in New Territory* in 2000, I have learned a great deal about being a self-published author. This third edition is, to my eye, flawless. I hope you will find yourself and your family in these pages. But especially yourself.

INTRODUCTION

This handbook is designed to be a "quick read." When your brakes fail on a steep mountain road, you probably won't reach for your 400-page owner's manual to determine what to do next. You need driving skills and you need them fast! The current books on Parent Care contain excellent information on what to do for your parents, but limited practical guidance on how to keep your emotional balance as adult children.

Here we are in our fifties or sixties; our children are raised, and the grandchildren are brilliant. Our careers are at a place where we can begin to embark on the dream of increased leisure time. Then the phone rings: Dad has had a stroke. In a flash of thirty seconds, we are thrust into role reversal. This is a *rite of passage* we are not prepared for, even if we knew it was inevitable.

Most of us have good coping skills. As adults, we have learned to deal with marriage, divorce, children, stressful work situations, illness, success, failure; all the things that "grown-ups" are supposed to know. What baffles us is that our adult coping skills don't work very well when we apply them to our families. We find ourselves mired in old feelings, new guilt, and conflicts with siblings that have not happened since childhood. We struggle to find new ways to communicate with people who are now looking to us for guidance. Set a boundary with Mom? Share the load with Sis? I can't do that!! You can, but it has to be done with finesse and love. This golden rite of passage can be viewed as a time to grow into our sense of self, as that self relates in a new way to our parents and siblings.

When we were children fifty years ago, families naturally absorbed relatives who outlived the actuarial tables. Many of us grew up in small towns with social systems we could count on. Social Security was a new concept, and Medicare did not exist. Family was the center of our social and influence circle. Today, in our fast-moving urban/suburban, Internet-surfing, Mars-exploring world, families are separated by geography and lifestyle. For most of us, the way our parents took care of Grandma no longer works. What is the new model?

The new model is born of population density, mobility of the nuclear family, affluence, and longer life spans. At this moment in time, the new face of aging in the twenty-first century is developing, but what will the final picture look like?

Assisted-living centers and retirement communities

are springing up like mushrooms in winter. Are these the answer? Partly. We are transitioning from the caregiving models of our childhood. Facilities with porticoes and elevators represent the "big house" where Great-Grandmother lives today. Our grandchildren won't sing "Over the river and through the woods, to grandmother's house we go" with the same mental pictures we have. We are stepping into a new territory, but we are poised in mid-air, unable to keep the commitment to the old ways and unfamiliar with the new. Our discomfort is understandable. All these new ways to be old are a stretch for us.

Adult children are forging new territory. We live in a time when people are deemed "old" in their late eighties and nineties.

Many of our grandparents died in their sixties. We may have a photo of our grandmother in "old lady" shoes, hair in a bun at the nape of her neck, an apron covering her dress. She was reflecting what society expected a grandmother to look like. She was probably 55! Think about what fifty and sixty look like in 2004: Goldie Hawn is 57. Vanessa Redgrave is 66. What about the guys? Al Pacino is 63. Sean Connery is 72. It's a new world!

Our parents are children of a yesterday we can hardly imagine. Most of them were born in the early twentieth century. What was it like to be a child in 1915? What was it like to be a teenager in the roaring twenties? What was it like to live through the Great Depression, and then in the next decade to experience the rationing of basic foods and fuel to support a world war? I have no memory that even comes close to that kind of fear or sacrifice.

We experienced the Korean and Vietnam wars, but there was no "war effort." Families watched the Vietnam war on television. Sacrifices of huge proportions were asked of the men and women who served, but those at home were observers, not cheerleaders. The reach for outer space that propelled technology and product development at breathtaking speed happened when we were young adults, and are part of our life experience. My father, on the other hand, told of arguing with his siblings to see which one of them struck the match that lit the taillight on their first automobile. We live on the same planet, in different worlds.

As we struggle with the extreme difference in life experiences, we should remember that our parents formed values and grew to be adults in a world where change was catastrophic. They had to trust those around them and conform to their community standards or risk being ostracized. To be ostracized in their world could be life threatening. To be nonconformist in our experience is just another life choice among many life choices.

It is helpful to "walk a mile in the shoes" of your parents. Where did they grow up? If it was rural Iowa, the structure of their life is very different than if it was the lower West Side of Manhattan. What has been their relationship with money? How do they view authority? Are the police always right? Is the doctor all-knowing and never to be questioned or confronted with errors in judgment? Older people love talk about the old days. Let them share, and use their information to walk that "mile in their shoes." This won't guarantee that the challenges of caregiving will never be frustrating, but you will be able to understand why your parents see their world through the filter of a life experience that is vastly different from yours.

For the purposes of this handbook, the term "caregiver" applies to a wide range of activities, from long-distance "check-in" phone calls and two visits a year, to sharing a home with a parent and being the sole caregiver. Your caregiving might include arranging home care for parents in California while you live in Minnesota, or hiring someone to relieve you on a regular basis while your parent lives in your home.

As a caregiver, you may be feeling grateful to give back to your parent all that he has given to you. But you are just as likely to feel resentful and grumpy. Your feelings today are the result of a lifetime of interactions with your parent. Often the feelings are conflicted; there is the mixture of love and resentment, of anger and patience, the satisfaction of helping and at the same time feeling overwhelmed at what has been heaped upon you. All of this is perfectly natural and normal.

This handbook is not designed to help you resolve any of those feelings. It is designed to help you cope with the results of those feelings, and keep them from crushing you. Help with the deeper issues can be addressed in support groups or with a therapist. For example, the question "Why can't I say 'no' to Mom?" may be answered by finding small ways to start saying no, setting aside the underlying issues until you are less vulnerable. If you are currently in therapy, you and your therapist can best estimate your strength. We are encouraging your healthy passage through this phase of your life.

As we examine the adult child/ parent relationship we are going to assume that the aging parent has his or her cognitive skills more or less intact. Parents may be unreasonable or demanding, but they will respond to your behavior changes. They may not like it, but they will understand it. The excruciatingly difficult caregiving for dementia will be discussed in Part Four of this handbook.

As with any life challenge, there is a way to meet caregiving challenges with tools that work, as opposed to feeling broad-sided with each new crisis. Many of us are "clueless" about how to take care of ourselves as we become caregivers. We have all seen the angry, tight, sometimes frantic faces of adult sons and daughters as they accompany their parent in supermarkets, doctor's offices, and restaurants. Without saying a word, they seem to be shouting, "I am overwhelmed!" We must find ways to provide our parents the help that is needed without being so stressed ourselves that we miss the life lessons of the experience. There is a maturing, a seasoning, a deepening sense of self that happens as we find our way through the maze of conflicting emotions that surround an aging parent.

There are scores of books to guide us toward services that are available for our aging parents. We can do all the research needed to handle their medical, legal, and financial needs. But how do we manage a job, marriage, our children's needs, go to a movie, or take time to read a good novel? The information that follows may give you some ideas.

I describe a wide variety of coping skills in this handbook. The banquet table is set. Take what appeals to you and leave the rest. Come back for another look. Then take some more.

A NOTE TO
"FIFTY-SOMETHING" BABY BOOMERS

Mom and Dad are healthy, happy and doing just what you want to be doing when you're their age. Still, you're dreading what is going to happen to your life when the first major incident of decline happens. Or, perhaps there are a few health issues, but you are nowhere near the role reversal stage of the aging process. Now is when you need to read this book. Learn the skills, set the boundaries, visit an Elder Law attorney and get things into place while your parents are part of the decision-making process. Denial is your worst enemy. I can't tell you how many people have said to me, "Where was this book when I needed it?" Or, "I wish I had known this ten years ago." This book will give you a fighting chance to live your own life as you lovingly care for your parents in their declining years.

PART ONE

Where Do You Fit in Your Parents' Lives?

1

IF IT'S NOT BROKEN, DON'T FIX IT!

A young Japanese woman commented that American elders stay active and independent much longer than do Japanese elders. When I asked about this, she said that Japanese elders are made weak and dependent by having too much done for them. It is their cultural expectation that, at a certain age, their family cater to their every need. This may sound nice, but the end result is that the elders lose their self-confidence and independence.

In contrast, remaining engaged in life can have the opposite effect. An article in the *Wall Street Journal* (5 Aug 97) detailed how we should begin to plan for a second career by age 45. When retirement comes, the next phase of our working lives should be ready to roll. If we wait to make plans until right before retirement, it could be too late. We might have to go fishing or play golf instead of pursuing new vistas!

Do not create dependency. It is a serious mistake. When

a person is 75 years old, he may be that age on the outside, but from his eyes looking out, he is 45. He sees himself as capable of running the New York marathon. He may be correct. There is an entire senior division in the marathon. The title of a wonderful book on growing older by Walter M. Bortz, M.D., says it all: *We Live Too Short and Die Too Long.* Celebrate independence for your parents. Unless they are in physical or medical danger, don't interfere. Love them, spend time with them, and enjoy them.

If your parents are living independently with proper nutrition, safety, and strong social contacts, but you would like things to be 'better for them' in a retirement community near you, first ask them if they want anything to change. Older people abhor change. They like their neighborhood, even though you may think it has declined. They know their neighbors and the clerks at the grocery store. They may have purchased their gas at the same service station for forty-five years. Your convenience and your peace of mind is not of major importance here. Theirs is.

2

WHAT IS THE PROBLEM AND WHO IS IN CHARGE?

One of my favorite stories is a perfect metaphor for what we are about to explore. My husband and I were attending an engineering conference in Minneapolis. As a side trip, we visited the Northwest Airlines Flight Training Center. Our guide was a retired veteran pilot who had flown every type of airplane in every conceivable capacity, from open-cockpit mail delivery to senior pilot of a 747. Someone asked him, 'What was your most frightening experience?' He told us the story of flying a four-engine propeller plane. One of the engines flamed out on take-off. In the chaos that followed, the cockpit crew managed to kill two of the other engines. Everyone in the cockpit was taking control, and they nearly died as a result.

In the debriefing, the crew realized that they had not taken the necessary moment to assess the problem and assign the duties that would lead to a solution. To this day, 'What is the problem? Who is in charge?' are the first questions all Northwest pilots are trained to ask in any emergency. When you are confronted with a complex situation in your life, they are very good questions to ask yourself. Parental relationships can be very complex situations.

My father presented me with my first complex caregiving problem. As a terminal cancer patient, he was getting progressively weaker, spending most of his time in bed. He was living at home under hospice care. Household tasks had become too much for him. I suggested he hire a housekeeper. He tried someone for two weeks, didn't like her, and rejected any further help.

When the house deteriorated to unacceptable levels, I recommended someone come in for a few hours at the end of the day to tidy things up and get dinner ready. He said he would think about it, but never would agree to the help. Finally, I said, 'You are getting too weak to be here alone. If you don't get help, you will not be able to stay home.' I allowed two days for him to consider the 'ultimatum.' I had no power to force him into a nursing home, but I tried the threat anyway, and it worked.

I knew that staying home was my father's deepest desire. I wanted to honor his wishes, but knew his safety and well-being were at risk. I kept his freezer stocked with soups, stews, and other easy-to-eat home-made meals. I was a frequent visitor, but I was unwilling to be his in-home caregiver since he was more than capable of paying for one. It was a boundary decision I made when he was first diagnosed with lung cancer. I knew I was dealing with a 'black belt' controller.

My father's need for control was greater than his desire for help. When he finally accepted help, he was too physically weak to do anything else. He called the shots from the moment of diagnosis through his death. Calling the shots was the way he lived his life. It should have come as no surprise that he would orchestrate his death in the same manner. Who was in charge? He was. I could make suggestions, take him on tours of assisted living centers, worry about him, complain about his intractability, but ultimately I had to come to terms with the fact that he was going to do exactly as he pleased. He went to a skilled nursing home *three days before his death.* He did it his way.

⌒

Nancy, a member of an Adult Children of Aging Parents (ACAP) group, came storming into a meeting one night, so angry she could barely speak. Her mother was cared for by an agency nurse who was very invested in keeping his job. When it was time for hospice to be called in, the nurse told Nancy's mother, 'You don't need hospice, I can take care of you.' He saw hospice as a threat to his nursing assignment, when in fact, agency and hospice nurses are accustomed to working together.

The nurse didn't seem to understand that hospice is for

the entire family. Volunteers become part of the care team. Nancy needed the help offered by hospice volunteers, who would drive her mother to medical appointments, run care-related errands, and stay with Nancy's mother while Nancy rested or left the house for a few hours. Financially, she and her mother needed the free medication and medical devices that come with hospice care. The nurse convinced Nancy's mother to refuse the hospice program. The nurse was a major problem.

The ACAP group suggested that Nancy contact the physician who had ordered the hospice services. She did. The doctor made room in his schedule to see Nancy and the nurse the next day. The matter was settled in minutes. Hospice visits began. Nancy was exceptionally kind when requesting that the agency send a different nurse. She talked with nurse's supervisor, saying he was an excellent nurse, but that he needed some training in the areas of detachment, codependency, and the value of partnership between agency and hospice nurses. In this example, the problem was the nurse, and Nancy was in charge.

The dynamic between a trained caregiver and a client can be magic. One of my clients, a lady of ninety-two with early dementia, posed an extremely complex problem. She was evaluated for adult foster care by a geriatric care manager, and was deemed capable of remaining at home with the support of in-home care. Her only son and his wife were planning a trip out of the country for four months, and if my company was going to be responsible for her health and safety during their absence, all of us had to be certain home care was the best answer.

In the beginning, the client resisted any help. She was locked in a power struggle with her son, which only succeeded in making her more resistant. We tried three caregivers before we found the right personality match. Then, along came Mary. She has developed a relationship with the client that the son has never seen between his mother and anyone else. In fact, he is a little miffed. 'How come Mom wouldn't do that for me?'

The truth is, the right caregiver can perform 'miracles.' They don't have a history. There are no family 'pricklies' they have to overcome. When the right personality match is found, the results can be life-altering for everyone.

Wisely, the son had started looking eight months before his extended trip to find the best care situation for his mildly demented mother. The son had the guardianship. He could have placed his mother in foster care, but he wanted her to have the chance to stay at home if *she could cooperate with a caregiver.* Her stubbornness was not a trait born of dementia; it was lifelong personal style. Her son was in charge, but he handled his power with wisdom. Had we failed to find anyone to break through her resistance to help, the only answer would have been foster care, as she was not managing the tasks of daily living on her own. Because of her son's foresight and the way the caregiver has won cooperation from the client, the mother's independence was honored, and her health and safety were secured.

⌒

One of my favorite clients is a 101-year-old woman who is definitely in charge. When I met Mrs. C., she was being discharged to her home from a rehabilitation facility. Until she experienced a problem with her hip, she had been living alone in her well-maintained home, handling her own finances and reading a book a week. Her mental status cannot be questioned. Her 82-year-old son wants her to be in "a home" with around-the-clock care. Mrs. C. doesn't need that level of care. She agreed to wear a Lifeline for her security when she is alone, and that seemed to reassure her son. We have a caregiver with her four times a week to grocery shop and prepare meals and handle any tasks she may have for us. She has a housekeeper once a week. There is no reason for her to be in a higher level of care, or to be "hovered" over by daily caregiving. Who is in charge? She is. Being 101 years old does not make her incapable of living life on her terms.

3

STEPPING IN
WHEN THE ISSUE IS
HEALTH OR SAFETY

If you attend an Adult Children of Aging Parents meeting anywhere in the country, you will hear half of the participants describing their frustration about not being able to get their parents to accept the help they need. Everything they need could easily be obtained, but the parents refuse all suggestions.

This is a terrible position to be in. It is nearly impossible to walk away from a stubborn, demented, or dying parent *who must be helped.* You need to step in, but how do you do it? There are several directions to turn to for help. Your choice depends upon what you or your parent can afford to pay for the help. Money determines the resource you use, not the result. There is always an answer.

One of the answers that fits every budget is embodied in a new specialty in the legal profession called Elder Law. Elder Law helps the low- to moderate-income elderly meet their care cost needs by gaining access to public benefits.

This field of law grew to address the unmet needs of people who were unable to navigate the complicated statutory schemes established to gatekeep the various healthcare payment programs.

Elder Law works for the woman who spent thirty years on the line at Heublein Corp. making sure the mustard jars were properly filled and who now lives on a small, fixed income and has acquired a modest savings. Her medications are so expensive that regardless of how well she has planned for her old age, she will run out of money long before she runs out of life. And yet, she has too much money to qualify for assistance under the Medicaid Program.

An Elder Law attorney will be able to provide solutions, often in the form of specially-crafted trust documents, that will legally bring the woman's resources and income within the Medicaid means-testing guidelines (as those guidelines are applied in her state). Once she is eligible for Medicaid services, she will have access to all of the Medicaid benefits. All she really needs are Medicaid-supported prescriptions, but access to this benefit is only available to those who (1) meet the means-testing portion of the Medicaid guidelines and (2) demonstrate a need for care. The Elder Law attorney will assist with the financial aspects of the case, and an Elder Law social worker will evaluate the healthcare needs.

An Elder Law social worker might establish this woman's eligibility for home care at three hours once a week, for a month. After that entry into the system, she will qualify for all Medicaid services. Even though all she needs is help with her prescription costs, prescription help alone is not a doorway into the system. The easiest access into the system is through a minor amount of home care.

As a result of the attorney's help, our mustard lady's ongoing financial needs will be handled out of her trust. With the hundreds of dollars she saves through government-subsidized prescriptions, she can now pay her car insurance, buy food, and go to a movie once in a while. The government wins because Medicaid is not tapped for all her needs. Our mustard lady wins by remaining independent. She lives on an allotted portion of her income (a community-based care allowance) and a special-needs trust established for her benefit, while using the public system only for her major area of need. Before Elder Law, she would have gone through virtually all of her money, jeopardized her home to medical costs and become completely dependent upon the government for medication *and* housing, food, and medical care. Medicaid is a convoluted system, but it is accessible with professional help.

Another specialty of Elder Law is to establish a durable power of attorney for finances and advance directive for healthcare and place them in the hands of competent and loving children long before they are needed. My 92-year-old client signed a power of attorney agreement that established her son as her financial agent-in-fact when she was in her early seventies. She trusted him to act in her best interest when and if she was no longer able to care for her finances. (Perhaps she knew her stubborn nature would get her in trouble one day?) Whatever the reason, her son would not have been able to enjoy his retirement without that legal power. He knew he might look forward to twenty or thirty years of taking care of his mother. The power of attorney and advance directive for healthcare assured him that he would be able to handle her finances and personal care without outside intervention. We must understand the importance of negotiating the proper legal controls when they can be done by agreement, not by a judge declaring our parent incompetent. That is a horrible process for everyone.

Elder Law offices are staffed with social workers and attorneys who work together to 'negotiate the eggshells' of helping parents see the wisdom of planning for potential issues well before they are needed. Emotion can stop people from making good decisions or even suggesting that good decisions be made. Elder Law professionals do the reasoning with the parents, so the children are not seen as vultures awaiting their parents' deaths. This sticky situation requires training and experience to navigate. It's a pretty good bet that if you can get your parents into an appointment with Elder Law specialists, they can handle the rest. Choose carefully, interviewing attorneys before you bring in your parents. You need to feel confident that they can help you. You may only have one chance.

Whether your parents are applying for Medicaid or

Medicare benefits, you'll face the inevitable bureaucratic paperwork. After approval of benefits, Medicaid recipients have less red tape because they are issued a card to use when they receive services. This is not so with Medicare. If you have dealt with Medicare, you've seen bureaucracy at its worst. Oceans of paper lie between your parent and the medical care that doctors and hospitals would like to provide. It must be the belief of those at the federal Department of Health and Human Services that a Medicare patient knows how to swim through the never-ending streams of paper generated by benefit managers. Almost no one actually receives his or her maximum benefits. Elder Law attorneys will help your parents fight these systematic battles with Medicaid and Medicare. There are many ways in which these attorneys and social workers can help you as you care for your parents. Put away your lawyer jokes, and try them. You will receive more than you can imagine from this dedicated group.

Another little-known resource is the Area Agency on Aging. It was created by Congress to establish a local resource for the aging and their families. They provide information and referral for senior housing, caseworkers to follow clients in their search for financial assistance, transportation, legal advice, counseling and support, caregiving, housekeeping services, meals, home repairs, financial subsidy for food and medications, senior centers, and protection from abuse. Their services are provided on a sliding-fee scale. Everyone is eligible.

The Area Agency on Aging is not as visible as it should be. Most people think it is a county office that's just for the poor. Not so. I've found them to be wonderful, devoted people doing a great job. Utilize this exceptional product of your federal and local taxes to support you as you walk the road of weary caregivers.

4

WHERE IS
MARCUS WELBY WHEN
YOU NEED HIM?

I love the story of the old man who went to the doctor complaining he had a pain in his right knee. The doctor said, 'Oh, that just happens when you get old.' The man replied, 'That's funny, the other knee is the same age, and it doesn't hurt at all.'

Taking your parent to the doctor can be an experience fraught with frustration. There are multiple reasons for this, all of which we will discuss, but there is one parent/ doctor issue that needs to be understood, because it will not change. We grow up with a set of values and beliefs, which replicate those of our communities. With few exceptions, our parents were brought up to trust authority. They have a difficult time believing that a president would lie, that a policeman would be brutal, or that a doctor may not know what he is doing. It is a core belief. When your parent does not question a doctor, even when a vital symptom has been missed, the wrong drug used, or medical neglect has led to the death of a loved one, it is because 'the doctor knows what he is doing.' When we understand this mind-set, we can work around it.

A good way to work around this core belief is to gather information from our parents about their pain, movement difficulties, and sleep or eating pattern changes. We can take them to their doctor appointment armed with a written list to guide the doctor's observations. Set the stage by saying, 'The doctor wants to know what is happening with you. We both know when he comes in and asks how you are, you will say, 'I'm fine.' I am going to give him a list of the problems you've been telling me about. Doctors today are very busy and won't take the time to question you. If all you say is 'I'm fine,' he will accept that, pat you on the head, and you will still be in pain. It's not like the days when Doctor Williams came to the house, took care of us, then stayed for dinner.'

When you acknowledge that your parent's 'I'm fine' comes from a core belief that the doctor is all-knowing, it will be much easier to help them communicate appropriately. This will make you and your parent allies rather than adversaries. If you are living six thousand miles away and are doing your symptom questioning over the phone, call the doctor's office, get the fax number, and send the list of concerns via fax. I can't tell you why, but doctors will read a fax whereas they may not look at a letter or promptly return a phone call. Keep a copy of the symptom list for future reference should the problems not be addressed or resolved.

Unfortunately, the medical profession has experienced some profound changes in the past ten years. The consolidation of professionals into an HMO system plus a reduction in Medicare benefits has made older patients' access to medical treatment more difficult. The time physicians have to spend with their patients, particularly Medicare patients with low reimbursements, is limited. They are under the gun to get in and out of the examining room with lightning speed. This does not describe every doctor, but it describes too many.

Helping your parents to choose the right doctor will reduce your stress level. Geriatric specialists are the best choice for our parents. The number of geriatric specialists is not growing at the same rate as the senior population. Even though it may seem difficult to get an appointment with one of these doctors, it is worth the wait. They can diagnose in spite of vagueness on the part of their patients. Geriatric specialists understand that old age is not an illness to be cured, but a stage of life that requires specific treatments. Because babies can't tell a pediatrician what is happening to them, pediatricians are trained to read signs and symptoms. The same is true for geriatric specialists. Understanding opposite ends of the life cycle requires good detectives.

Family practice physicians would be the second-best choice. Internal medicine physicians would be my last choice. IMs are good doctors, they are just too busy to take the time needed for the elderly. And many clinics that do not have a geriatric department limit the number of Medicare patients they will accept.

⁓

The Medicare caps came to my attention when one of my clients' daughters called me in a state of fury. Her mother was a patient at one of the city's larger medical clinics. The daughter was not happy with the internist her mother was seeing and wanted to change doctors. She was told that none of the established internists would accept a new Medicare patient. She responded by saying, 'All right, forget Medicare, she will be private pay.'

The answer was, 'I'm sorry, those are the clinic rules.' The clinic was not going to assign one more time-consuming elderly patient to a busy internist. The mother could see their newest physician, who still had time on his schedule. The daughter said, 'No thank you. My mother does not want a doctor younger than her grandson.' The doors to the clinic were shut to a woman who had been its patient for sixty years! I referred my client to a geriatric group. There was a three-month wait, but it was worth it.

⁓

This is a good point to take a little side trip to discuss Medicare. When I worked as an intervention specialist at a medical center in California, we had a patient whose drinking had rapidly progressed into alcoholism following his retirement from a major bank. His insurance provided full coverage for in-patient treatment of alcoholism. But because he had applied for Social Security benefits, he was automatically enrolled in the Medicare system.

Medicare became his primary insurance. Under Medicare requirements, he could not be admitted to alcohol treatment because he had not *failed* at two prior forms of treatment. Catch 22. His insurance from the bank could not override Medicare, so he wrote a check for treatment. There is something wrong with this system. Why Medicare is not means tested is beyond understanding. If my patient had insurance that would pay for his treatment, he should have been able to use it. It is my hope that the 'protest problem-solving style' of the baby boomers will change this state of affairs when they find that their private medical coverage is of little value. This is the end of my political bandwagon speech.

If your parents are in an HMO, ask for what they need, and don't stop with the first person who puts up a roadblock. The elderly need a physician who is a geriatric specialist. Some elderly need geriatric psychiatrists to evaluate dementia and prescribe medication to relieve the symptoms of the many forms of this devastating brain disorder.

As an example, my mother had Alzheimer's disease.

When her geriatric psychiatrist managed her treatment, things went very well. But when her medical doctors prescribed medications, paying only cursory attention to her existing medication list, she became a mess. I finally left an order at the Alzheimer's unit that no medication—prescription or over-the-counter—was to go into my mother's mouth without her psychiatrist's approval. The medication nightmare ended. My mother stopped experiencing drug-induced problems until the very end, when everyone dropped the ball. I describe this in chapter 20.

Manage your stress level by learning a little 'doctor talk.' Many large hospitals have a health/medical library that is open to anyone who wishes to use it. The helpful librarians will know what you need and where to find it. Educate yourself enough to be able to ask questions that will make the doctor listen to you. You need to know how your parents' medications work so you can discuss them with the doctor. A doctor is a human being, one who is probably a little disappointed that his profession has taken such a quality nose-dive. Help him or her to be a good helper for your parent. When you visit the doctor with your parent, take along the list of questions and symptoms you wish to discuss. Don't leave until you are satisfied that you have been listened to. Don't allow a doctor to get away with the 'That's just part of getting old' routine. That is too easy, and not acceptable.

Nurses are a wonderful resource. Nursing managers of the medical/ surgical floor at local hospitals are good people to help you find a physician. They know all the good ones, *and they know which ones to avoid.* How do you get a nurse to make a recommendation? You ask her to have a 'non-conversation' with you. You talk about your difficulty in finding a physician who does not think your parent is a throwaway person. She will help, then swear you to secrecy.

Geriatric nurse practitioners (GNP), geriatric clinical nurse specialists, and social workers can be a huge help in assessing the condition of your parent and directing you to the medical and in-home help that you need.

Have a GNP look at all of your parent's prescription medications, over-the-counter remedies, *and* vitamin supplements. A primary care physician is expected to carefully monitor your parent's overall care. It's a nice idea, but it doesn't usually happen. Your parent may be seeing three or more doctors, with medications being filled at several pharmacies. When one doctor doesn't know what the other is prescribing, a problem with drug interaction can happen. GNPs can tactfully talk with the physicians and get orders to discontinue unnecessary or dangerous medications. Many elderly will continue to take a medication forever if it is not discontinued. The entire medication picture needs to be monitored closely and frequently.

You can find these professionals through your state nurses' association or under Geriatric Care Managers in the Senior Services listings of the phone book. (See Part

Five for telephone and Web site information.)

Geriatric care managers can be nurses or social workers in private practice, or groups of professionals working as a team. GCMs are trained to look at medications, mental acuity, physical signs and symptoms, physical surroundings, current level of care—all the things that make up the overall well-being of your parents. If in-home care is needed, they tap their pool of privately contracted caregivers or engage a service such as Home Instead Senior Care, which staffs quality, bonded and insured caregivers. GCMs will work with your parents' physicians, often placing pressure on them to fill your parents' needs with results that you could never achieve on your own.

One of your largest caregiving challenges is to advocate for your parents in the often frustrating arena of medical care. The more you know, the more you will be heard. The better the choice of physician, the better the quality of care. You can reduce your stress by being informed and assertive.

There is hope and help on the horizon. Dr. Welby is making a come-back! In recent years a national organization, the American Academy of Home Care Physicians, has been formed to promote the art, science, and practice of medicine in the home. Physicians can be found who make house calls and care for homebound patients. Why is this happening? Doctors are frustrated with a medical profession run by insurance companies whose only interest is minimizing the cost of care. Cumbersome as it is, Medicare does not second-guess the physician in the same manner as an HMO. Many home-care physicians are specializing in problems of the aging.

I am delighted with the quality of care my clients receive when they receive home visits. In Portland there is a group of doctors and geriatric nurse practitioners with the company name, House Call Providers. I have nothing but admiration for doctors and nurses who have begun to think "outside the box." Walking into a patient's home can tell the doctor volumes about the patient's condition. Are your parents safe at home? Ask the doctor. She was there yesterday. How do you find home care physicians in your area? Email: aahcp@mindspring.com, look them up on the web at www.aahcp.org, or pick up an old fashioned instrument called the phone and call them at 410-676-7966.

5

WE CAN
NEVER BE A PARENT
TO OUR PARENTS

Even though it may sometimes feel as though the parent/
child relationship has been inverted, any attempt to take
the role of the parent is to invite a power struggle. Our
parents will always see us as 'the kids' even though we may
be sixty years old. It is frustrating, but that is probably the
way it is in your family. If you have been fortunate enough
to develop an adult-to-adult friendship with your parents,
they may be able to hear you without resistance when you
make suggestions about the decisions they are facing. But,
more commonly, your parents may listen to a complete
stranger before they will listen to you. The supporting and
caregiving role is difficult, even with perfect parents. Do
you know of any?

We know what doesn't work in these relationships.
There is a way to map this new territory so our children
will have a model to follow. As mature adults, if we want
the relationship with our children to be less combative

when we are old, now is the time to make changes. If you have children over thirty, they are adults. Stop treating them like children. This is the time to become adult friends with our children. How do we do that?

Look at the relationship with your best friend. How do you talk with him/her? Do you share your feelings? Do you tell the truth? Do you refrain from telling them how to run their life unless they specifically ask for your advice? Do you know you will lose their friendship if you behave horribly to them?

Stop being a parent and be a friend. Your children are always going to be part of your life; why not make it fun to be with them? The absolute cut-off date for telling them how to run their lives is thirty. Try it.

My children call to talk things over with me. They trust my judgment. They know a good way to solve a problem is to discuss it with three people they trust, think about what they heard, then make a decision that works for them. I am happy to be one of those three people once in a while. They don't always take my suggestions, but I don't always take theirs.

I know adult friendships can exist between parents and children. I saw such a friendship between my mother and my grandmother. Mom duplicated that relationship with me. I will never forget picking her and Dad up at the airport after an extended trip to the desert. I found Mom at the luggage carousel and gave the usual 'How was your trip?' greeting. She said to me, 'If I were ten years younger, I would see a divorce lawyer tomorrow.' That is not the usual parent reply. The usual parent reply would be: 'We had a lovely trip, darling.'

My mother and grandmother were my teachers, and my children are the beneficiaries of their lessons. My children are capable, bright, interesting people, and I take great care to treat them in that manner. When I don't, they are quick to remind me to 'bug off.'

It is possible to develop adult-to-adult friendships with aging parents, but it's not easy. If your parents are able to talk about feelings, able to share what's really happening in their lives, you may be able to get around the 'me parent, you kid' roadblocks. Be cautious with aging parents. Be open with them, but don't give them information that will worry them or keep them awake at night. If you've never had a real conversation with your parents and the door begins to open, go slowly. Don't tell them their favorite grandson got arrested for marijuana possession and you were up half the night at the police station. You may understand the 'rite of passage' of a teenager butting heads with the legal system, but Grandma and Grandpa will build that into a term in prison, with their darling grandson consorting with dope addicts and drug dealers.

It is never too late to try to be your parents' friend, but don't be disappointed if it doesn't happen. Do what you can do. Concentrate on seeing that the next generation relates to you differently before you are old.

6

COULD YOUR PARENTS
NEED PROTECTION
FROM YOU?

Let's stage an example of how this can happen. Imagine that your mother died two years ago after a lingering illness. Dad went on a cruise to the Greek Islands with a group of his men friends, and while on board, he met a woman. He came home acting like an eighteen-year-old, excited and happy for the first time in years.

This scene could play out in two ways. You could throw a fit, refusing to ever speak to your father again if he continues with this impulsive relationship and attempting to convince him the woman is probably after his money. Or, you could keep all your protective thoughts to yourself and share in his happiness. At the same time, the investigation you requested from the Pinkerton Agency might reveal that Dad's friend is a lovely lady of impeccable reputation, who is also financially independent. Whether she is right for Dad is for him to determine.

If we wish to live our lives on our terms, we must have

the same respect for others, including our parents.

The frail are the ones who lose ownership of their lives. I made a blunder with my mother and learned a lesson I can pass on to you. My mother had Macular Degeneration, which left her unable to see what was directly in front of her. Alzheimer's disease had destroyed the link that sends messages between her hand and her brain. So, lipstick became an issue. Mom was uncapping the lipstick, rolling it up too far, breaking off the stick, and getting lipstick all over herself, her bathroom, and her clothes. I was putting away garments in her closet when I saw the lipstick disaster one time too many. I gathered up the lipsticks and asked that the aids handle them in the future.

Anticipating that Mom would be upset, I had a very logical and loving way to explain the problem. I was going to appeal to her lifetime sense of beautiful grooming and explain that she could not be expected to see the lipstick when her central vision was gone. Wouldn't it be better to have one of the staff help with the makeup?

It turned out that Mom agreed: lipstick was a problem. She agreed that the staff should help her with lipstick. What she objected to was that I made the decision to remove the lipstick without talking to her about it. I was completely wrong and agreed to be more respectful in the future. Because so much of her life had been taken away by her vision and memory loss, she needed to be consulted on anything where she still had some control. I had walked all over the little control she still had in her life.

A common caregiving mistake is overprotection. I got a call from a woman concerned about her sister. The sister, age seventy-two, was bright, capable, and energetic. But her sons were undermining her confidence by being overly protective. They cautioned her not to drive into the city because there was too much traffic for her to cope with. One son built a 'grandmother' addition to his house for her to move into so he could take care of her. The sons were at her front door if she didn't answer the phone. She felt smothered, diminished, and incompetent. She had difficulty telling them to back off because she knew they meant well. And, after all, now that she thought about it, maybe she was 'losing it'?

My caller said that her sister was fabulous. She did not need driving help. She did not need a place to live where someone could take care of her. She was perfectly capable of taking care of herself in her lovely condominium. She needed protection from her sons. As a solution, I recommended that she contact a therapist I know in her community. The family needed some counseling. The sons didn't sound malicious, they just didn't understand the harm they were doing. With help, they would see they were killing their mother's spirit and confidence. She needs the freedom to do what she wants to do, go where she wants to go, and live where she wants to live. There are years ahead for her to live a full life.

It is useful to look at the above example from another

angle. What do we call the husband who tells his wife she is incapable of handling the checkbook? He tells her she can't go visit her mother out of state because she would never make it through the maze of the airport. He calls her five times a day to check on her whereabouts. If you have watched this kind of behavior, you know it is called emotional abuse. Only the strongest egos are able to sustain mental health under this kind of continued diminishment. Is there really a difference between this husband and my caregiver's nephews? The husband is an abusive controller, and the sons think they are taking care of their mother. The result is the same. Both lose their self-confidence, believe they are defective, and begin to disappear into a shell of depression and despair. Adult children need to be aware that overprotection can be as damaging as no attention at all.

A recent incident in my life illustrates how confidence can break down as we age. My husband expressed a concern about my safety when I drive at night in the rain. He said he saw things I didn't see (trucks? cars? cows? Who knows?) My response was, 'Thank you for sharing, but I will continue to drive at night until something happens to convince me to do otherwise.' We negotiated. Now, when we go out together at night, he drives. I bought new glasses to reduce the glare of oncoming cars and rain reflection. I told him his concerns were appreciated, but that overprotecting a 59-year-old woman was a downward spiral we did not need to ride. It is too easy to believe that we are over the hill when the first challenge of aging arises. We are a long way from that. Erosion of confidence happens insidiously.

What would have happened if I had agreed not to drive at night in the rain? My husband would have organized his schedule to be my driver. This is the trap of overprotection. If you protect too soon, you may find yourself appointed to a job you don't really want.

PART TWO

*Boundaries Are
the First Line of Defense*

7

SETTING BOUNDARIES: A COPING TOOL

Creating boundaries is a concept that is a little fuzzy around the edges for most people. Seldom do we have a good working definition to guide us. Here is the best one I have heard: A boundary lets me decide how far someone gets to come into my life.

We draw boundaries all the time. It is usually in our best interest to keep our personal life away from the workplace, so the place we are most likely to set boundaries is at work. People we work with are usually acquaintances rather than friends we have learned to trust. Many of us have worked with people who are like an open book. Most often their "book" contains information that pushes people away, interferes with their promotions, or brands them a loose cannon. We have good reason to be cautious about people who have no personal boundaries: they will not respect ours! They are intrusive without being aware of it.

We also draw boundaries when a friend is requiring more time, energy, or patience than we are willing to give. If we are no longer comfortable in their company, we become unavailable by saying, "I'd love to do it, but I just can't work it in." When this happens often enough, the relationship will be moved to a distance we can manage. This can be sad and we can have regrets when it happens, but for whatever reason, the relationship has changed. There is no longer space for that person in our life. I heard someone say once, if everyone who came into my life stayed in my life, it would be too crowded. Life is like a dinner table. The chairs will always be filled, but those who sit in the chairs may change over the years.

8

WHY IS IT SO DIFFICULT TO SET BOUNDARIES WITH FAMILY?

With whom are our relationships the most difficult? Who has the ability to inflict wounds that can take a lifetime to heal? Who are the "them" we refer to when we say, "Why can't I just spend time with them without always being on guard for land mines?"

The answer is, our families. We rarely, if ever set boundaries with our families, yet we are confounded when they seem to have the ability to turn our lives around on a dime. We appear to be perfectly happy to gift-wrap our lives and give them to the first family member who asks. For whatever reason, we are more likely to set boundaries with siblings. They don't seem to have the power of spouses, children, and parents.

We do not set adequate boundaries with family for one of two reasons: self-induced guilt or the external fear of "What will people think?" We all know people who never speak to their families. It appears that it is easier to erase

family from our lives than to deal with them. Why is that?
I don't believe we even consider that we have a right to set
boundaries with family—"After all, they are family." We
not only have a right, we have a responsibility to allow
our family members to be subject to the same criteria as
anyone else on this planet.

Setting boundaries with aging parents may be a daunting challenge if we did not create a natural break between
our parents and ourselves when we reached our early thir-
ties, or when our first child was born. If you haven't created a healthy distance between you and your parents, start
with small changes. A boundary that is set with kindness
and a smile lays down the line with invisible ink. As an
example: if Dad criticizes you unkindly or treats you like
an employee who is held in low regard, respond by saying, "You seem to be having a bad day today, I'll come by
another time." Smile and leave! Or, on the phone, say, "I'll
call you when you are feeling better, bye." Politely hang
up. Your dad may be startled, but do that consistently and
he will alter his behavior toward you. He wants your presence in his life. You may not change his basic disposition,
but he will learn to be careful how he deals with you.

One of the hardest lessons I learned as an adult was that
I am a player in every relationship I have. This includes
my relationship with family. No one *makes me* angry, hurt,
or frustrated. *My response* to their behavior *causes me* to be
angry, hurt, or frustrated. Who controls how I respond to
my world? I do. I am 100 percent in charge of the inside of
my head. There are times I am perfectly capable of anger,

I can feel sorry for myself or strike out in frustration just like anyone else. However, it does not take me very long to decide that I am not willing to give away my head, rent-free!

Sometimes the lesson to be learned is so clear we can't avoid seeing it, even if we want to. The difficulty in setting boundaries with our families is vividly illustrated in the following stories, which give concrete examples of how those boundaries can be set. One of them may give you insight as you struggle with a similar problem.

9

THEY HIT THE
BOUNDARY WALL!

There are times when we need to set a boundary by saying no to an unreasonable request, or staying home when we know we need rest. It is not selfish to take care of ourselves. A caregiver with no personal boundaries, who functions with knee-jerk reactions to every demand, is too tired, angry, and resentful to be loving.

⁓

Marcy's parents had been married for fifty-nine years. Mom had suffered a stroke and needed to be in an assisted living facility. Each Sunday, Dad would bring Mom home for the day. Each Sunday would end in arguments and criticisms. Marcy stopped by twice for Sunday visits. She did not go a third time.

Dad complained about the Sunday "nightmare" each time Marcy talked to him. She would point out that he was the one who drove the car and made the Sunday plans. She strongly suggested that he not bring Mom home. Each time he did, she went through the grief of the loss of her home. She wasn't able to do the things she used to do. Dad was baffled that she could not enjoy their Sunday visit without a teary scene. Mom was hurt by his lack of sensitivity, but nothing changed. Finally, Marcy suffered her dad's complaints for the last time. She told him, "You keep setting this up. Don't do it anymore. Go to a movie, go for a drive, go out to lunch; *do anything,* but don't go home expecting everything to be like it used to be."

Mom was terribly hurt by Dad's behavior. She kept bringing it up over and over with Marcy. She didn't think she could say no to the Sunday ritual. Marcy finally saw it was fruitless to discuss the problem with either of them. Her parents continued to put themselves through the same ringer for two and a half years! Trying to change the patterns that had developed over fifty-nine years of marriage was too much for them.

Listening to their complaints was making Marcy crazy. Marcy set two boundaries. One: She refused to listen to her parents complain, because neither of them was willing to change the situation. Two: She did not go anywhere near her parents on Sunday. They had the right to make each other miserable. She did not have to join them. She continued to visit with them individually. She hated to see this happening to them, but she had done all the counseling she was willing to do.

Sally's mother had been in an excellent nursing home for five years. A series of increasingly severe strokes had left her verbally nonresponsive. No one really knew if she was able to understand what was going on around her. Was she locked in a body that could not respond? Sally was going to the nursing home every night to feed her mother.

Sally's husband had recently retired from a successful career and wanted to travel and spend time at their home on the Oregon Coast. He wanted to play golf with his wife on warm summer evenings. Sally couldn't bring herself to do any of these things if it meant leaving her mother for even a day, although she was getting excellent care at one of the best nursing homes in the area. Sally's mother had been an independent, powerful woman in her healthy years, and if she were able she would tell Sally to "get a life." But Sally feels her responsibility toward her mother requires sacrifice.

How could a good, Catholic girl like Sally expect to behave differently? She couldn't, until she got permission. How did she do that? Sally began attending a regular group meeting of Adult Children of Aging Parents (ACAP). Through the group process she began to see what she was doing to herself, her marriage, and her health. Most importantly, the group gave her permission to reexamine her current relationship with her mother. Her daily visits came out of guilt, not the actual needs of her mother. Of course she cared, but Mother would not go without her dinner if Sally was not there. Sally set a small boundary. She would not go to the nursing home on the weekends.

Her next step was to plan a vacation with her husband. She hired an outside caregiver to visit with her mother while she was away. Even though it was a wonderful nursing home, Sally wanted to be sure her mother got focused attention on a regular basis. Hiring the caregiver may seem unnecessary, but it was an effective way for Sally to assure herself that if Mother *was* locked within that body and aware of her surroundings, she wouldn't feel abandoned. Sally will always be a devoted daughter. That is who she is. She is attempting to create a balance between her devotion and her own life. That is a healthy boundary.

It is much easier to set a boundary with a physically passive parent than it is to come face to face with a parent who resists any change you try to make. The fear of setting boundaries and the parental reaction that a boundary may create keep us in jail even when we have the key in our hands.

⌒⌒

Anna lived with her mother who needed help, but wasn't helpless. Mom was an overweight diabetic who'd lost her lower left leg due to circulation problems caused by remaining overweight and not keeping her insulin in a control zone. Anna belonged to an ACAP group. She described her mom as controlling, demanding, and nearly impossible to live with. She would come to group appearing on the edge of emotional collapse.

One night Anna announced to the group that she had found a new job, her dream job. She was energized for the first time in years. Like so many of us, Anna had slowly given away her life because she was strong and capable. Only in looking back can we see the extent to which we have been captured by being strong and assuming the role of "taking care of things."

The ACAP group knew enough about the dynamics of Anna's family to recognize that the new job was a perfect opportunity for Anna to begin to change patterns and set boundaries. It only took six weeks for the inevitable crisis to happen. Anna was no longer coming home for lunch every day. She took several business trips. Mom was losing control, and she didn't like it. When a huge scene occurred, the family doctor was called in to referee. He'd been trying to get Mom to take antidepressants for years. She had refused. The doctor was concerned about Anna's health as well. He told Mom that if she didn't improve her horrible disposition, Anna would walk out. He would see to it!

The group members could not believe Anna's face when she walked into the next meeting. She looked ten years younger! She and Mom had both been prescribed new generation antidepressants and had attended their first family counseling sessions. *The crisis had persuaded Mom to take the medication she so desperately needed.* Anna's use of the antidepressant was situational. She would undoubtedly function well without it when her life stabilized. In eight

weeks, her mother had gone from "a mother from hell" to
a cooperative roommate.

The real tragedy in this story is how different Anna's
and her mother's lives might have been, had Mom been
treated for depression years ago. It is exhausting for those
who suffer from untreated clinical depression to try to
live a life that resembles what they think life should be.
If one is clinically depressed, it is impossible to "pull it
together."

The magic of that particular ACAP meeting wasn't
over. A new woman had joined the group and described
a situation that was just like Anna's. We all looked at
Anna, who had begun laughing with tears running down
her cheeks. She told the new woman, "I need your phone
number. I can save you a lot of grief."

Anna's story illustrates three important points. First:
Stay alert to an opportunity to set a boundary. Second: *A
crisis is not a bad thing. It can rapidly change family patterns.* Finally: *The group magic does happen.* Anna, who had
been emotionally battered by her mother for years, listened
to the suggestion of the group, and within months her life
was turning around. She could then give her experience to
a newcomer, thus passing on the wisdom of the group.

Sandy intentionally distanced himself from his family. He
moved from Seattle to Fort Lauderdale, Florida, at age 18.
He moved as far away as he could get and still stay in the

continental United States. One sunny February morning forty years later, his phone rang, and he heard the weak, little voice of his 84-year-old mother on the line: "I've had enough of this rain. I am moving to Florida."

Sandy had always been pleasant to his mother, remembering birthdays and Christmas, making phone calls a couple of times a year, *but he really didn't like her.* Panic hit the moment he hung up the phone. He couldn't forbid his mother to live in Florida. What if she wanted to live with him?

Sandy called his friend Jerry, the caregiver of an aging parent. Jerry took Sandy to an ACAP group the next night. The group did some emergency "coping-skill" training with Sandy, and he began to feel safe. He wisely rejected the idea that his mother come live with him. He helped her select a retirement community where she could go on with her life in a milder climate. After all, this was her stated purpose for moving to Florida.

Sandy set a clear boundary with his mother from day she arrived. If she called to ask for something, he would say, "Let me think about it and call you back tomorrow." Or, "Let me look at my schedule and get back to you in a little while." He may have been perfectly happy to run an errand for her, or come for dinner, but he would not say "yes" instantly to anything. He was training her that a knee-jerk reaction was not going to come from him. He gave himself time to think through any request, regardless of the urgency she placed in her voice. This boundary helped Sandy remember that every demand didn't represent a crisis; his mother was living in a retirement community specifically chosen to support her health and safety.

This is not a happily-ever-after story where mother and son are reunited. Sandy didn't find that his mother had magically turned into a nice person. She was someone he would be cautious with were she a neighbor or a co-worker. He chose to have a cautious adult-to-adult relationship with her, being kind, polite, and pleasant, but not emotionally vulnerable. Sandy did what he knew was the "right thing"—being kind without seriously altering his life. Had he not understood the importance of the "never say yes immediately" boundary, he would have had a daily struggle to retain a balanced life. He made the decision as to how far his mother was to be allowed into his life.

⁓

Janet's mom was a lifelong complainer who found all her attention needs met when she was ill. Mom lived alone, didn't keep her doctor appointments or take her pills carefully, and periodically went into a medical crisis, requiring that Janet drop everything and get her to the emergency room. After the crisis, Janet would do home care for a few days.

The ACAP group helped Janet look logically at her mother's life patterns: *Mom knows how to get attention. She creates a crisis. Janet jumps in and gives her all sorts of attention.* Negative reinforcement? You bet. The group suggested that the next time this self-inflicted crisis happened Janet call 911, and let the paramedics deal with

Mom. She will only have to do that two or three times, and Mom will start keeping her doctor appointments and taking her medication properly. Janet may catch her mother's wrath, but she can point out to Mom in a calm, nonjudgmental way that she creates the crisis through her own neglect. Mom has a choice and so does Janet. But if Mom continues the self-destructive behavior, Janet can choose to manage the crisis by calling in the paramedics. That is a boundary.

The other side of the behavior change is that Janet now plans enjoyable events for her and Mom. They go to a play or movie, take the children shopping, even travel together to another state to visit family. Mom may learn that her need for attention does not have to be crisis driven. Janet is careful to remember that her mother views life as a struggle and is unlikely to change that life script.

The adult children in each example found a way to be supportive to their parents, and at the same time set boundaries that allowed them to take care of themselves.

We can set boundaries with our families in small increments. Don't think a small step is unimportant. Think of the pilot who alters the course of his cross-country flight by one degree every hour. He will be a long distance from where he would have landed had he remained on the original course.

This whimsical definition of stress describes how easily nice people can lose control of their lives: Stress is what happens when your inside voice is screaming, "I can't do this" and your mouth is saying, "Of course, I'd be happy to..."

10

"SHOULD" IS
A RED-FLAG WORD

Just in case you were wondering, this is a section on GUILT. The word "should" is your signal that the thought running through your mind is driven by guilt. Guilt affects how you understand and react; it is like seeing an event through an unfocused lens. The lens distortion is the guilt. Guilt distorts the truth of a situation.

It is an inalienable truth that the person to whom an outcome is most critical should take charge of achieving that outcome. Don't take responsibility for something that matters a great deal to someone else, but is of little consequence to you. If you choose to go ahead, and you fail, don't accept the guilt. I will give you two scenes to illustrate this point.

Your mother has been given a medication that will make her "loopy" until her body adjusts to the presence of the drug. This will only last a couple of weeks, but she will be at risk of falling or bruising while she is off balance. On the way home from the doctor, you reiterate the doctor's warning about the unsteadiness she is going to experience. You strongly suggest that a caregiver be hired for this short period of time. She resists. You point out that if she falls, she may not be able to get up on her own. You remind her of Aunt Lilly who fell, was on the floor for two days, and not only had a broken hip, but got pneumonia because she was cold and couldn't move. Your mother says, "You and your sister can check on me, it will be fine."

You respond, "No, it will not be fine. I'm going to be out of town on business, and Kate is in Palm Desert for the month." Your mother huffs a bit, as she remembers your sister is gone and is put out with you for having a schedule that does not work well for her. Again, you bring up the caregiver. This goes on and on with no resolution. She refuses to consider outside help, even for two weeks.

Six days later, your mother falls and shatters her shoulder. She is in the hospital, and you are in Los Angeles on a business trip. Your guilt is overwhelming: "I should have insisted Mother have a caregiver. I should have canceled my trip and stayed with her. I should have called my cousin in Fresno to come up and be with her for two weeks. I am a terrible daughter. My mother will never forgive me. *Mother's broken shoulder is my fault.*"

You didn't do something you believe you should have done. Subsequently, something negative happened, and you assigned yourself responsibility for that new problem.

Here is another example. Let's take this to an everyday occurrence. You put a load of clothes in the dryer for your teenage daughter. Your daughter is getting ready for school the next morning and can't find her favorite pants. They were left in the dryer overnight *and they are wrinkled.* She is furious with you. You should have remembered to set the buzzer. You should have remembered to take the clothes out of the dryer last night even if the buzzer didn't go off. You shouldn't have fallen asleep watching TV when there was work to be done for your family. Guilt is dripping off you. *Her wrinkled pants are your fault, and you are a terrible mother.*

Again, you didn't do something you believe you should have done. Subsequently, something negative happened, and you assigned yourself responsibility for that new problem.

Let's look at both scenes of this two-act play. What is really happening here? In scene one, your mother is a 72-year-old woman who has been healthy and independent until this current problem. Many issues are layered here. This is your mother's first age-related health crisis. It is understandable for her to be resistant to outside help. She knows she is going to be off balance and at risk of falling, but nothing bad is going to happen to her, she is sure of that. Nothing ever has.

Your mother sees you as "her child." Your opinion is no more valuable to her today than it was when you were seventeen. You intuitively responded in an appropriate manner to her statement, "You and your sister can look in on me." You and your sister have your own lives. You have healthy boundaries. You need to keep them.

Your mother refused to accept help. She fell. The responsibility is hers. You did everything you could do. You cannot force someone to do what is good for her unless she is incapable of making decisions for herself. Your mother is not incompetent. Her denial and pride cost her months of pain. She made the rules; the consequences are her responsibility. If you are unwilling to soak up the guilt she will attempt to pour on you because you were out of town, you will give her the opportunity to be accountable for her actions.

Now, to the second act. Your daughter is seventeen years old. Where is it written that you are responsible for her laundry? Even if you know her clothes are less likely to color-bleed if you sort and wash them, she can certainly take them out of the dryer and hang them up. There are many layers to this scene as well, and you know what they are. She will never grow up if you don't give her responsibility for her clothes, her homework, her behavior, her friends, her spending money. You can begin this process by suggesting that she look in her closet for the clothes she wants to wear, and if something isn't there, to look for it or choose something else.

There is a familiar prayer that covers this two-act play: "God, grant me the serenity to accept the things I cannot change, the courage to change the things I can, and the wisdom to know the difference." You could not have changed your mother's attitude if you reasoned with her for twenty-four hours straight. You can change your daughter's household responsibilities, if you are willing to take the flack she will throw at you because you expect her to do something.

When a situation arises and you start "shoulding" on yourself, analyze what's going on. Can you do anything more than you have done? Is this really your responsibility? Can you do anything at all to make the situation different? Go back to the Serenity Prayer. It will help you decide whether or not to take responsibility for what is being asked of you.

〜〜〜

Everyday events can be barbed guilt hooks. A caregiver I interviewed told me that she had to have a minimum of thirty hours of work, each week. I explained that we match our caregivers to clients by personality, availability of the caregiver to work the hours requested by the client, and geographical proximity. I could not guarantee her thirty hours a week. There were too many variables to consider. She seemed to accept that. Then the phone calls began. "I have to have work. I can't pay my rent. You need to get me assigned to clients right away." I suggested that she register with several caregiving agencies, which would increase her chances of getting work. She said, "No, I only want to work for you."

I pointed out that she was placing herself in a no-win position. I was happy we had made such a positive impression on her, but I was not responsible for her rent. This lady was trying to dump her life in my lap, and I wasn't going to play. She was very pleasant in her interview, her references were good, and her background check was clear, but I will never put her to work. She is a proficient guilt spreader. My clients are vulnerable to sad stories, and she could easily take advantage of their soft hearts.

There are a lot more guilt provokers than responsible people in this world. Pay attention to what is said around you. When you react to a sad story and feel you should save someone from their problems, look out for that red-flag word.

I experience guilt infrequently. I say that this is because I am too selfish, but there was an instance where guilt had me, and I had no idea how I was going to work through it.

I was at an Alzheimer's support group, and I told the group, "It is so difficult to visit my mother. The person I have known and adored all my life is not there. She only knows who I am for a few seconds; then, in her eyes, I morph into her sister or one of my daughters. The only way I can communicate with her is through music. She can't complete a thought, but she can sing an old song. I turn on the music and sing with her. She looks at me and says, 'You sing just like my daughter.' It breaks my heart."

The group facilitator said, "Don't go." I was stunned. She asked me if my presence was making my mother's life better. Was I a comfort to her? Did she depend upon my visits to take care of things she couldn't handle? Did she miss me when I wasn't there? I answered, "It used to be that way. She used to tell me she didn't know what she would do without me. But now, most of the time she speaks in a language no one can understand. She does not remember that I was there five seconds after I have gone."

The facilitator said again, "Don't go." That was impossible for me to contemplate. I was overwhelmed by guilt just at the thought of how nice it would be to stay away.

Quite accidentally, I found something that helped my mother and did not require me to visit as often. My husband and I were visiting one day and we sang to her. She was thrilled. Later that week, the Alzheimer's unit called to ask me if I had a tape of my singing, or Bud and I singing. They thought it would have a calming effect on her when she was agitated. I had done a tape of lullabies for my grandchildren. It was sung as if I had a baby in my arms, very quiet, very soothing. I took it to Mother and it had a magical effect on her. She knew my voice, and it was as if I was there singing to her. She would listen for long periods of time with her eyes shut and a smile on her face. My voice could soothe her when she was screaming and no one knew how to help her. Of course I continued to visit, but not as often as I once did. I was there at the touch of a button on a tape recorder.

When I am doing what is right for me, I am doing what is right for everyone else in my life. That sounds selfish, but it isn't. Never underestimate the most powerful societal constraint of all, "What will people think?" Adult children slip easily into guilt when they dare to take care of themselves first. Do dare, you deserve it. If not you, who? More about that in Part Five.

11

CONTROL CAN BE
AN OLYMPIC EVENT

Aging people are likely be controllers even if that was not
their personal style in younger years. It is understandable.
Their entire lives are out of control. Their bodies don't
work like they used to, their minds may not work like
they used to, their health is failing, their friends are dying,
their spouse of a lifetime may have died. These are frightening events, and the need to control what is controllable
is natural. Have you ever been to an assisted living center
when the dining room staff is ten minutes late opening
the doors? It is not a pretty picture. There is a mini-riot
in the hall. The time of the meal is one of the few things
the residents can depend upon. Everything else on their
agendas, including medications, may vary, but never the
dining room hours.

This is a good time to strongly suggest, NEVER set a
predictable schedule of visits to your parent. It is a control issue, and you can keep your parent from being upset

by not setting expectations. Traffic happens, unscheduled appointments happen, life happens. If you are expected at 3:00 and you arrive at 3:45, your mother may have decided you are dead on the freeway, neglectful, or both. It is better to call right before you arrive to be sure she is home, than to be expected and late.

Control happens in many different disguises. People control the actions of others through:

Anger	Power
Weakness	Fear
Money	Addiction
Silence	Illness
Pity	Chronic lateness
Guilt	Non-stop talking

These twelve styles have variations and are seldom as cut and dried as the list would imply. For example, power can mask as leadership, silence can mask as passive aggression, and addiction can mask as something as benign as an inflexible exercise schedule.

Learn to identify the control styles in your family. There may be as many styles as you have family members! The best defense against being controlled is to recognize it when it happens. As a training exercise, watch what happens at the service desk of a local auto parts store or the lost luggage counter at an airport. Watch people at a large table in a restaurant. Who controls the situations, and how do they do it? Start paying attention to strangers, then coworkers, then friends, then yourself—then family. By the time you get to your family, you will be an expert.

I have a friend whose brother is chronically late. It's his way of keeping people off balance. It is a subtle but effective control style. Being keenly aware of her brother's control style, my friend made a decision to work around it. She invited him to dinner at 6:30. At 6:00 she and her husband had a hearty snack of cheese and crackers as they settled in to read their e-mail. Her brother arrived at 7: 45. They didn't ask him about heavy traffic. They weren't upset and annoyed with him. They welcomed him, poured him a glass of wine and sat down for a leisurely chat. She had identified his control style and made a conscious decision to love him as he was.

Ask your friends to help you see your personal control style. If you are like me, you learned your style from a parent. I know my control style is power. The use of power to control others got in my way often enough that it caught my attention. Therapy resolved a great deal of the problem. I am a natural leader. The right use of power is in that context. But when I turn the amps up and try to power my way through a situation, I recognize control rearing its ugly head. It is amusing to see how I react to someone who is behaving as I used to behave. I have this urge to wring their neck until I realize where this unreasonable thought is originating. It used to take hours, even days for me to

recognize this "reflection" reaction. Now is only takes seconds. Practice does help.

"Control" controls us when we are unaware it is happening. There is infinite freedom in side-stepping control.
It is important to recognize the control style of your family
so you can identify that knot forming in your stomach as
something that has little to do with you and everything to
do with the person who is attempting to control you.

I laughingly refer to my franchise, Home Instead Senior
Care, as a "rent-a-sibling service." This nickname came
about when I was interviewing the mother of an exhausted
only son. She was reclining in her bed with "the vapors."
For those of you who are too young to know about the
vapors, it describes a lady "taking to her bed" with some
unknown ailment that requires her to get a lot of attention!! I chatted with the prospective client for a few minutes, then began to describe our services. Each time I said,
"Our caregiver can..." she would interrupt with "Phillip
can do that." Finally, I said, " Mrs. D., your son is an only
child with a busy life. His family understands his devotion
to you, but they need time with him too. Phillip is going
to rent a sister." She thought about that for a few minutes
while both Phillip and I were smart enough to keep quiet.
At last, she said, "I guess that will be all right." And it
was, until she sabotaged it. Her need to control was stron-
ger than Phillip's ability to set a boundary.

My father was tall, good-looking, charming when it
suited him, wealthy, and formidable. He gifted varying
amounts of money annually to my brother and me, our

children, and his sisters. If I had told him his gifts were a form of control he would not have the vaguest idea what I meant. He thought the gifting came from love, and in many ways it did. But the underlying motive was control of his family.

When two of the grandchildren did not live up to his expectations, he ended their annual $10,000 gifts. That was the moment I made the decision to walk away from the money if I could not outmaneuver the controlling. It was interesting to watch his reaction the first time he threatened to cut me off because I opposed him. My response was, "It's your money, give it to the Salvation Army." It took a while for him to understand that I meant what I was saying, but he did finally get it. As a result, we had a delightful relationship, and the gifting continued.

I did not change my father's behavior, except as it applied to me. I decided how I was going to respond to the control. I was not willing to live with the constant self-monitoring that trying to please a controller always creates. Did I out-control the controller? Probably.

An amusing moment came of all this. My mother asked me with some awe in her voice what I had done to my father. It seems he was talking to her about me, and with a little smile on his face said, "I'm not going to push her around, she scares me." That was wonderful news. I had that big bear just where I wanted him.

We are unlikely to alter anyone's overall control patterns. What we can do is decide if we are going to allow the control.

12

LOOK BEFORE YOU LEAP: CAN YOU SHARE A HOME WITH YOUR PARENTS?

Before you make a decision to live with an aging parent, you must ask yourself some questions. The most important questions are: Do you have a balanced life? Can you say no?

A balanced life includes:
- a strong social system of friends, two or three of whom you can always count on to be there for you;

- a career and/or volunteer work that gives you a sense of accomplishment and self-worth;

- a hobby or activities that give you pleasure and challenge your intellect;

- exercising regularly and eating in a manner that supports your health and well-being;

- entering into intimate relationships—when you
  do—because they nurture you in some way, and not
  just out of convenience;

- a strong spiritual connection to God, as you understand God to be.

Can you say no? Personal boundaries are intricately tied
to being able to say no. If you have boundaries, you will
be able to say no when you mean no, and yes when you
mean yes.

If you are considering sharing a home with an elderly
parent, make an agreement with them. Put the agreement
in writing before you make the move. Consider the following points:

1. Determine how the house is to be divided. Each person
   must have personal space that is open to the other by
   invitation only.

2. Allow that whoever owns the home is in charge of the
   home. (If the carpets need to be cleaned, it does not
   need to be a committee decision.)

3. Decide how the household responsibilities will be divided. Even the very frail need to feel they can contribute,
   no matter how small it may seem.

4. Talk about everyday preferences—leaving lights on or

off, television use, making the bed, putting down the toilet seat, how the phone is answered, etc. No detail is too small on a preference list. It's the little things that will drive you crazy.

5. Decide on a financial plan. Who pays for what? How is the money combined?

6. Agree to put in place a power of attorney for health and finances that will allow you to help when your parent cannot make good decisions. (If this is impossible, the whole idea may be impossible.)

7. Openly discuss the inevitable role reversals and agree, in writing, to seek counseling should a power struggle begin. Agree upon how the cost of counseling is to be shared.

8. Agree to hire respite care when you need time away from home. You must be able to get away from each other on a regular basis. A parent may resist in-home help by saying, "Oh, I'll be fine, don't worry about me." You will worry! Find a caregiver your parent will enjoy in your absence. Which one of you pays the caregiver needs to be negotiated as well.

9. Take your parent to retirement communities, assisted living facilities, and foster care homes before you make a final decision. There is always more than one

choice. Don't look back with the "if I had only known" regrets.

The final question to ask yourself is, *Is my intention coming from a willing heart or from guilt?* If the answer is guilt, go back to number nine. If you do decide to take the plunge, the book *What to Do When Mom Moves In* by Betty Kuhn can help. It covers all aspects of in-home parent care; see Part Five for more information.

PART THREE

Siblings: Part of the Problem
or Part of the Solution?

13

DON'T COMPETE —
COMMUNICATE!

Siblings cooperating to provide care and support for an aging parent can work together like a well-choreographed ballet. Unfortunately, that happens all too seldom. A more frequent occurrence is lack of cooperation, power struggles, or outright refusal by a sibling to be involved in parent care.

As an example, a local caregiver can be driven to thoughts of violence when an out-of-town sibling destroys the slow, painstaking progress he has been building with a stubborn parent. Day after day, the local sibling has observed the dementia and physical deterioration of his father. He has finally gotten Father to agree to move into an adult foster home with around-the-clock care, good food, and secure surroundings. When the out-of-town sibling arrives, Father pulls himself together for the duration of the visit. The out-of-town sibling sees his father functioning just fine. Obviously his brother is overreacting. A huge argument occurs within Father's hearing, and all the groundwork that was laid is instantly destroyed. The out-of-town sibling leaves, and Father drops back to the lower level of functioning.

What the visiting brother did not know is that a person with dementia can seem completely normal one day, and the next day accuse a caregiver of stealing all his clothing. It is a disease of paranoia, delusions, and missed perceptions. With dementia, there are good days and bad days. There is something about a visit from a seldom-seen child, sister, or old friend can bring about the ability to "pull it all together" for a brief period of time.

The lesson is: If you are the local caregiver, communicate. A great deal of pain can be avoided if the out-of-town "hero" arrives and supports your efforts. The visiting brother in the illustration above really thought his father was being "put away in a home" by his overreacting brother. Had he been made aware of the increasing symptoms of dementia that had necessitated the move to full-time care as they were occurring, he would likely have supported the idea. The reverse is also true: If you are the out-of-town sibling, ask a lot of questions before you dive in and interfere with the plans that are being carefully set in place by your local brothers and sisters.

14

FALLING INTO OLD BEHAVIOR PATTERNS

Under the stress of a family crisis, particularly the illness of a parent, siblings often revert to old behavior. Perfectly mature, centered adults can dissolve into rivalries they have not experienced since they were ten years old. This can be very disconcerting. You feel as though you should look in the mirror to be sure you are still there.

"I can't believe how I behave when my sister is here," said a very centered, 55-year-old friend of mine. Her mom had broken her hip. The two sisters were trying to problem-solve Mom's future. My friend described herself as taking a position that was in opposition to everything her sister suggested. I explained that families in crisis often revert to childhood patterns of interaction. The old "Mom loved you best" jealousy or the "lost middle child" abdicating responsibility to the others is not uncommon. Family crises and family celebrations tend to bring out old behavior.

Sibling relationships during caregiving can be dicey. Don't assume that because you have a common problem you will instantly become comrades in search of the best for all concerned. Step back, look at your siblings. Ask yourself some hard questions. What is the history of the relationship? Do you trust this person? Are you emotionally safe if you share your deepest feelings? Will your sibling use your vulnerability against you? Does your parent play one of you against the other? Is one of you looking for the best doctor to insure your parent's well-being while another is working with a lawyer to secure his inheritance, and another is planning to move to the other side of the country?

With each sibling going off in a different direction, the end result will be chaos. One way to contain the chaos is to "assign" each sibling to do what he is going to do anyway. Those who want to distance themselves can send money! Grit your teeth. The brother who is consulting the lawyer will seem benign when you thank him for looking into this difficult problem. Anger and resentment will cause more stress than accepting what you cannot change.

We, as capable adults are still "the kids" to our parents. The CEO of a major corporation is a kid to his parents. In an aging-related crisis, the parent, who may have been the traditional family leader, is no longer able to assume that role—yet our ideas on how to proceed through the crisis hold about as much clout as they did when we were teenagers. Often when consensus has been reached and the siblings present a united opinion on what needs to be done next, a parent is likely to agree with minimum resistance.

This next story has nothing to do with adult children, but it is a perfect example of falling into old behavior patterns.

One of the most puzzling experiences of my life was attending my oldest daughter's college graduation. Her father and I had been divorced for several years. When our parents, our three other children, and the two of us sat down together for the graduation exercises, I felt as though the years of separation had never existed. We were a family. All of us were behaving exactly as though everything was normal. The kids wanted to drive Dad's new car, so for the ride back to the hotel, my ex and I drove their old college rattletrap car.

That was the strangest moment of all. For twenty years we had laughed about having four children in college at the same time and what that could do to our "comfort." Here we were in a car where you could practically see the road through the floorboard, living out the prediction, and laughing all the way to the family dinner. The only thing we didn't do was share a hotel room that night, although that crossed both our minds. When I described this bizarre scene to a therapist friend of mine, she said it was absolutely normal to have a major family celebration or family crisis wipe out intervening years.

As in the scene I just described, when you feel as though you are in a time warp, go for a walk around the block, hide in the bathroom, do whatever it takes to find a few minutes to reorient yourself. Remember who you are, where you are, and why you are there. Time warp is most likely to happen if you have moved away from your natal family and you are out of the "family patterns."

⌒

What's the best coping skill for a family crisis? If you find a knot forming in your stomach, or feel the early signs of a huge headache and all you want to do is escape, step back and look at what is happening around you. It is possible that by altering your behavior, you can alter the situation. One of my "stepping back and observing skills" is remembering that everyone around me is expressing a cry for help or an act of love. If I can stop reacting long enough to remember that, I can respond with kindness. I am aware that I am "making myself" act with kindness rather than confrontation. It is difficult to respond in the exact opposite of instinct.

The most exasperating people are the ones who are exhibiting their anger as a cry for help. If you told them that was what they were doing, they would accuse you of being out of your mind, but that's what is happening. These people don't want to be angry or alienate those around them. They think their only way of gaining attention is through negative behavior. The people who make you the craziest have limited self-esteem.

Only you can alter your attitude. You are responsible for what happens inside your head. You are responsible for your actions, reactions, and inaction. Unless you are dealing with someone who is in an advanced stage of dementia or suffering a severe character disorder, you can alter relationships by altering your behavior.

When you are having a bad day, isn't everyone around you irritating and difficult? The reverse is true. When you are happy and contented, everyone around you responds to your mood and they are all wonderful, too. Who sets that up? It's not "THEM." Monitor your thoughts. Refuse to invite the negative and angry thoughts to take your attention. Let them come in and flow on through. You may be surprised at what happens. Wouldn't it be wonderful if just by changing your attitude and behavior, you could be an adult friend to your sibling? "Oh, right, you don't know my sister."

Have I just read your mind? If I can read it, you can control it.

15

END THE GOOD KID/
BAD KID GAME

If Mom has always played one of you against the other,
that family dynamic is a control tactic every bit as effective as the wrist movements of a puppeteer. Don't expect
adult reactions to old childhood rivalries just because you
are 45 or 55 years old. If siblings can talk about what is
happening, the game may not stop, but the damage will.
Think how great it would be to have humor in your non-
verbal eye contact with your brother that says, "There she
goes again!" You and your sibling could be a team instead
of unwitting rivals.

In an ACAP meeting, Barbara discussed how she broke
up a divide-and-conquer game in a work situation that
later allowed her to defuse the good kid/bad kid game in
her family.

There were only three people in Barbara's office. Her
boss would tell her something and say, "Now, don't tell
Marion about this, but..." He would do the same thing

with Marion. Barbara and Marion would each hear a part of the information, but only the boss knew the whole story. They finally figured out what was going on and told the boss, "This is a very small office. We work very closely with each other. You need to know that what you tell one of us, you have told both of us. We find it is much easier for us to do a good job for you if we communicate openly with each other." They said it respectfully, but they said it, and it worked. The game stopped.

The game is unlikely to be stopped in a family that easily, but siblings can openly discuss the problem. Barbara described using her work experience with her brother. It took a lot of courage to name the problem, but she told him, "As far as Dad is concerned, you can't do anything right and I can't do anything wrong. That does not make it true, and it doesn't make it right. I know how valuable you are. Dad would be lost without you. We can't change him, but we can know that it has little or nothing to do with you or me. It is the way he sees his world, based upon his childhood experience with his father." That discussion healed a lot of pain for her brother. It was true, it had nothing to do with who they were, but everything to do with who Dad was.

16

WORK TOGETHER
TO BUILD CONSENSUS

I asked a hospice nurse to tell me her favorite "healthy family" story. She recounted walking into the home of a patient and being confronted by six very businesslike family members, four children and two spouses. They wanted to know where she went to nursing school. What was her GPA? How long had she been a hospice nurse? All this before she got past the entry hall. At first she felt attacked, but in a nanosecond of consideration she realized they were working as a team for the well-being of their much-loved mother. This group continued to work together, building consensus on even the smallest issues. The last months of their mother's life were not marred by family strife.

As I listened to this story I was reminded of December 1998 when my husband's sister suddenly died of a flu-induced cardiac failure at the age of sixty-two. Her three adult children were in close contact with us for a week. All of us were reeling from the tragic loss of such a vibrant presence in our lives. The children had problem-solved in a consensus model all of their lives. When it looked like the gathering after the funeral was going to be a do-it-yourself disaster, I came charging in and reserved a golf club dining room and catering staff, without consulting anyone. A family meeting was called and I was in big trouble. It wasn't that they objected to the plans, they just wanted to take part in the decision. My M.O. is to see something that needs to be done and do it. That is not the way to work with that type of group. I have every reason to believe that had my sister-in-law lived to old age, they would have worked together in sharing caregiving responsibility with nary a ripple in their family pattern.

When a family is scattered around the country, consensus and participation in caregiving is very important. Your brother in New York may be able to participate by sending money, which increases caregiving choices. Your sister in Florida may offer to have Mom come to stay with her for two months during the winter. Florida has wonderful resources for seniors to pursue friendships and entertainment. Your sister in Maryland who just retired, may offer to come home for a visit and spend the month giving you respite support. Your brother at Microsoft may surf the Net for resources for you. Ask for help. Most people want to help. They can contribute within the range of things they can reasonably do.

Some siblings refuse to help, even though their help is desperately needed. A startling example of sibling alienation occurred at an ACAP meeting in Portland, Oregon. A man came into the meeting, visibly shaking and obviously very upset. He placed a loaded gun on the table and announced, "I just left my mother at my brother's house."

He had been providing around-the-clock care for his severely demented mother. His brother had not responded to any of his requests for help. His brother was perfectly capable of helping, physically or financially, but refused to have anything to do with mother or her care. He had taken his mother to his brother's front door, placed the gun against her head and threatened to shoot her right there, on the porch, if his brother did not take her in. The brother opened his door and took his mother in.

The rest of the meeting (after the facilitator had secured the gun) was spent problem-solving the man through that evening and the next day. He was immediately put in touch with crisis counselors by cell phone. There was general brainstorming about community resources that were available for him and his mother. He did not even know that these existed. By the end of the meeting, he was calmer, mildly hopeful, and went home for his first uninterrupted night's sleep in two years. The following week Mother was placed in an excellent foster care home that specializes in dementia residents. But for that week, his brother was the caregiver!

This event was as severe a cry for help as any sibling can express. So much pain could have been avoided if the caregiving brother had been aware of the community resources available to him and his mother. If his noninvolved brother had done the same research the group did in a matter of two hours at seven o'clock at night, he could have helped his mother *and* kept his distance. Every family member can contribute at some level, but not every member will. Acceptance of your siblings as they are can keep your expectations realistic and reduce anger-based stress.

17

IF ONE PART
CHANGES, THE WHOLE
MUST CHANGE

A pie chart is an interesting metaphor for the family. We have all seen pie charts visually describe statistics. There is an absolute about a pie chart: If one part changes, the whole must change. If the segment that represents 22 percent suddenly is shifted to represent 31 percent, the rest of the chart has to realign itself in every area. If your family is the pie chart and you change the way you function within the family, your "segment change" will create change in the whole.

You have a powerful ability to effect change. If you have been the family "s—disturber," always causing contention, stop doing that. If you have been the family door mat, stop being that. Those roles cannot be changed overnight, but they can change quickly. Kindness is a wonderful tool to disarm those who have been cautious of you or vice versa. Even the small step of a 2 percent change in your part of the family dynamic will effect the whole. Your family is not immune to universal law!

18

A FAMILY
OF STRANGERS

Couples are remarrying in their fifties, sixties, seventies, and even eighties. The children in such *not-very-blended* families may see each other a few times over the years. They can be convivial, but few feel the need to be part of a working family. After all, they were adults with established lives when their parents married.

In an ideal world, when the parents become old and in need of help, the "strangers" who comprise these separate families would come together and share the tasks that create safety and well-being for both parents. In the real world, that may not happen unless the parents, prior to the inevitable incidents of aging, have done some serious planning.

What kind of planning can parents do? They can look at all of their adult children and assess them. Who can be depended upon to make good decisions about money management? Who would make a good advocate in issues of health care? Very quietly and in confidence, they can contact those children and gain permission to place these responsibilities in their hands when the time comes. The parents should meet with an attorney and get their wishes legally in place long before the first age-related incident.

Parents should choose by determining which adult child's lifestyle demonstrates which capabilities. Responsibility need not be based on age order, sex, or whose child is whose. When the first incident of aging occurs, will the children who were not selected have their feelings hurt? Probably. They'll get over it. They will quickly see that their parents have saved the family as a whole from experiencing destructive internal arguments in which no one wins and everyone loses. Those who don't get over it would have been the troublemakers!

When family battles occur at the bedside of an aging parent, they have little to do with what is good for the parents and everything to do with power, control, jealousy, and money. In some families where the adult children first meet at their parents' wedding and next in the hospital social worker's office, conflict may be impossible to avoid. In that case, parents who have chosen their representatives can rest assured that, if need be, the courts will back their decision about family leadership. Adversarial committees do not make good decisions.

What if none of the adult children are good candidates for family leadership? There are wonderful people called Guardian/Conservators and Geriatric Care Managers who can be hired to act in the parents' best interests. Parents who think power struggles between their children would never happen, blended family or not, should know that these two groups of professionals are available if war does break out. It might be a good idea to designate professional management from the outset if parents are overly concerned about hurting the feelings of their children.

A power struggle in front of aging parents is the most painful thing that can possibly happen. It is easy to prevent with some thoughtful advance planning. Ask your parents to help you avoid future problems by seeking the advice of an Elder Law attorney before the first incidents of aging. They may refuse, as though they can't conceive of any problems happening. Ask them to do it for the family. Ask them to do it for you.

PART FOUR

Where Did My Mother Go?

19

WHAT KIND
OF BEHAVIOR
CAN YOU EXPECT?

Our parents are who they are. Research has shown that human personality is formed before we are six years old. The bad news is, often our worst traits become exacerbated with age. Some advice you will see often in this handbook is to "have realistic expectations." I offer a story to illustrate the point.

A woman came to the gate of an ancient city and asked the gatekeeper, "What kind of people live in this city?" He asked her what kind of people lived in the city she had just left. She said, "They were selfish, horrible people who treated me very badly." The gatekeeper told the woman that the people in this city would be just like the ones she described and he doubted she would be happy here, so she went on.

A few minutes later another woman approached the gatekeeper with the same question about the city's

she had just left. She said, "They were selfish, horrible people who treated me very badly." The gatekeeper
told the woman that the people in this city would be
just like the ones she described and he doubted she
would be happy here, so she went on.

A few minutes later another woman approached
the gatekeeper with the same question about the city's
inhabitants. He asked her the same question about the
city she had left. She said, "They were all wonderful
people, happy and kind. I was so sad to leave. But I
knew that a new experience awaited me if I moved on."
The gatekeeper opened the door and beckoned her to
come in. "You will like it here, the people are just as
nice as those you left."

We receive from the world exactly what we project
onto the world, taking ourselves wherever we go, decade
by decade.

My daughter once tearfully asked me why she could
not talk to her father. She wanted gut level/feeling-based
conversations with him, and he does not "do" feelings. I
told her, "Think of your father as an oak tree. He is a grand
and wonderful oak, but don't stand at the base of that tree
and shout, 'You are a tree, I want apples!' Oak trees cannot
produce apples. No matter how badly you want him to be
an apple tree, it's not going to happen."

If your parents have responded to life as victims or
optimists, chances are very good they will end their lives
in a similar manner. There are always exceptions to this.

A transformational, life-altering experience can improve their life views, or a brain disorder such as Alzheimer's can remove a personality completely. Those are the extremes of possibility.

Try not to be overly concerned if your parents experience some memory loss. The aging process itself brings on forgetfulness. Having difficulty remembering can be likened to a computer process; the more data the computer holds, the slower the hard disk will retrieve it. Eighty years of data can clog the retrieval system. It helps to share the computer analogy when older people struggle to remember something. This can be very reassuring; they won't feel nearly as defective if a computer has the same problem they do!

Many older people are computer phobic. They resist using automatic teller machines. Try to get them through their resistance. Studies have proven that the mature brain continues to grow new neuron connections with each learning experience. Encourage the use of ATMs and debit cards at the grocery store. Introduce your parents to computer use by finding something compelling they will be fascinated to try. The longer we can keep their brains working with reading, listening to books on tape, going to senior centers to learn new art forms, dance steps, musical instruments, or even try the computer; the longer we will have them "present" in our lives.

When the brain becomes sluggish out of fear of new things, the person we know begins to disappear. If Mom has always wanted to play the piano, buy her a $200 keyboard with all the bells and whistles that will make her feel successful the minute she turns it on. She will think it's the lack of a huge piano in the living room that's been holding her back from learning. All she really needs is a lightweight, tabletop keyboard.

⌢

Don't be surprised if everything you do with your parent takes three times longer than you anticipate. One of the ACAP group members had us all laughing with heads nodding when she described a quick stop at her mother's house to bring her prescription refills. Her mother complained she was bored, so Lilly invited her to go to the grocery store, followed by a Starbuck's visit. Lilly geared down to her mother's slower pace through the store and coffee shop. The forty-five minutes had turned into two hours. Lilly had timed events based upon how fast she moves. All estimates were out the window when she added a vision-impaired, 83-year-old lady into the equation!

When I was on a tight schedule I didn't even consider stopping to see my mother. Dementia did not dim her perceptivness. She knew when I was rushed and not hiding my impatience very well. She may have been old and suffering from all sorts of serious defects, but she was still my mother and read me like a book.

It is important to remember that the natural process of aging will change our parents. If we are very lucky they will remain happy, energetic, and emotionally available to us until they die. But it is also possible they will be less energetic, grumpy, and become people we hardly know. We have a picture of our parents in our minds and hearts, and when that picture does not match reality it can be very painful. Getting angry with our parents because they are not what we want them to be is not useful, but it is understandable. When I became too overwhelmed by my mother's disappearance into dementia, I would get in the car and go hug a grandchild. As I touch their smooth baby skin and watch their endless energy, I know my mother was just like this eighty-two years ago. Life is a cycle, and the universe is in perfect order.

I had a little mantra that I said each time I walked into the Alzheimer's unit: "The light of God surrounds me, the love of God enfolds me, the power of God protects me, and the presence of God watches over me. Wherever I am, God is." I wrapped myself in a white light, took a deep breath, and opened the front door with a greeting smile for the nursing staff.

A woman who struggled for two years with the drastic irreversible changes in her mother as the result of a stroke, shared this insight that has changed her life: "I treat my mother as someone I have just met. She is now the nice lady who lives at my mother's house."

20

OLD AGE AND POST-TRAUMATIC STRESS DISORDER

As our parents age, their worlds become smaller. Older people talk about their bowel movements with the same interest they used to talk about their golf scores or their gardens. "Why does my aunt always talk about her health? Why are ailments the main topic of conversation with all her friends?" The answer to those questions is post-traumatic stress disorder (PTSD). Mary Pipher describes this phenomenon beautifully in her book *Another Country:* "Illness is the battleground of old age. It is where we all make our last stand. It is their World War, the Great Depression, and Hurricane Hugo. Like all PTSD victims, the old are interested in trauma stories. They talk to work through the trauma. They talk because health issues are the fast-breaking disaster story. Like other victims of PTSD, the old become obsessed with that which has traumatized them." *Another Country* is a must read for all adult children. It allows one to enter their parent's world.

For a moment, imagine you have survived a plane crash. You will talk about it for years. Repeating the story is the way your mind heals the trauma. Depression, obsessions, and addictions can be reactions to trauma.

I have a client who has been taking Valium since her husband's death. He died twenty years ago! Now, twenty years later, she is seriously depressed, as are many elderly, and the antidepressants are not working because the tranquilizers are offsetting the effect. She is taking two drugs that all but neutralize each other, leaving her "loopy" and sad. Her doctor's lack of prescriptive responsibility actually added to her distress.

Why does all the talk of illness tax the patience of adult children? Because most of us have the inner strength to "brush ourselves off and start all over again." It is difficult for us to identify with the battleground of old age. An aging woman who has broken a hip, learned to walk again, then suffers a mild stroke has very little inner strength left to draw upon. We can help older people build new strength by allowing them to process the trauma verbally without feeling they will drive us out of the room if they tell one more doctor story. Every one of us has the capacity to be a therapist. Each time we listen with empathy to the thoughts, feelings, and fears of another, we are being naturally therapeutic.

When family members begin to burn out, nonfamily caregivers can be magical healers. When a caregiver-client relationship is built on trust and mutual respect, the results are rewarding to family, client, and caregiver. Keep

in mind, caregivers do not have a personal history or emotional land mines to negotiate. They can sit and listen all
day. That is their job and they take it seriously. They are
trained to be therapeutic.

⁓

For example, I have a ninety-year-old diabetic client who
was suffering blackouts several times a month. Although
her blood sugar seemed to be in control, she would lose
consciousness, be rushed to the hospital, stabilize, and
return home. The client had moved from her home in
Florida to live with her daughter in Oregon. The move
itself induced significant stress. The daughter worked all
day. Mother could not be left alone safely, so I was called
in to provide a caregiver.

I will never forget introducing this client to her caregiver. She looked at this stranger in her living room and
asked, "Are you the one who is going to take care of me?"
The caregiver's answer was a stroke of genius. She said,
"No, we're going to be girlfriends." The energy in the
room shifted from resistance and dependency to one of
joy, and that is the way it has been since their first day
together.

My client has not suffered another blackout. She is
walking with new assurance, her eyes are bright, and her
humor has returned. She is a different person from the
fragile, withdrawn lady I met months before. The inner
healing we just discussed is happening. The relationship

between my client and her daughter has also improved with the caregiver's presence. So many of her mother's physical and emotional needs are met through the day that when the daughter comes home from work, there are cheerful conversations rather than complaints and problems awaiting her arrival.

An 86-year-old, retired RN told me, "I knew old age was going to be difficult, but I didn't think it would be this bad." And Oscar Wilde said, "The tragedy of old age is not that one is old, but that one is young." Old people want to drive their cars, go to the beach, wake up and hop out of bed feeling excited and happy. Sadly, those things are the memory of younger years. We can all cite exceptions, like the 85-year-old marathon runner or the 90-year-old man who goes to work every day to run his multimillion dollar business.

If you are ever in the Palm Springs area of California, don't miss the Palm Springs Follies. The cast of the Follies, all of whom are gorgeous with an average age of seventy, have overcome the ravages of age by taking exceptionally good care of themselves and placing themselves onstage. Imagine the condition of the muscles and bones of a dancer who joined the cast as soon as she reached the eligibility age of fifty! Granted, most of them have movie and theater backgrounds, but theirs is still an exceptional hobby. Sadly, most older people "resemble" the remark of Eubie Blake: "If I'd known I was going to live this long, I'd have taken better care of myself."

21

DEPRESSION: EPIDEMIC OF THE ELDERLY

Depression is the most underdiagnosed and undetreated ailment of the aging population. It is nearly impossible to have a gratifying relationship with a parent who is clinically depressed. Dr. Jeanne Jackson, a noted expert in the treatment of geriatric depression says, "The grumpy old men and women we all know are most likely suffering from untreated depression." It is epidemic in the older population. Dr. Jackson describes depression in a whimsical way by saying, "Imagine that we are all born with a full cupboard of green beans in our head. Throughout our life when a crisis happens we reach into the cupboard, open one of those cans, toss down the green beans, and everything levels out. Then one day we reach into the cupboard and there are no more green beans. Our natural equalizer is gone. Our usual way of reacting to life changes because we are missing an essential element in our brain. The antidepressant fills up the cupboard again."

For someone who is severely clinically depressed, suicide seems a good alternative. Dick Cavett, appearing on *Larry King Live*, described the depth of his depression with an unforgettable picture. He said, " If I was sitting in a chair across the room from a magic wand that would bring me everything I had always dreamed of, it just wouldn't be worth the effort to walk across the room and pick it up." No amount of self-talk or pep talks from others can bring a clinically depressed person back to the way they want to feel. They require medication. There are no more green beans in the cupboard.

A variety of new generation antidepressants work quickly and effectively. The old tricyclics such as Tofranil or Sinequan are rarely the drug of choice. If a physician prescribes them, question why. There should be some compelling reason to use the tricyclics. Often older physicians are not experienced with the new drugs and prescribe the old ones just out of habit or ignorance.

When an aging person is given antidepressants it is important to start with a low dosage and slowly increase to the normal adult dose. The older person's metabolism needs to be coaxed into accepting the drug. To start an elderly person on the adult dose of an antidepressant can make them drowsy and sluggish, and they may refuse to take it long enough to reach therapeutic effect. One bad experience with an antidepressant may make them negative about ever taking the drug again.

Talk with the doctor about your concerns over your parent and depression. If you are dealing with an internist, he may not be up to speed on geriatric medications and prescriptive dosing. It may be wise to lead him by suggesting a quarter-dose for a couple of weeks, then slowly working up to the full dose over a month or so. You can "help" by saying your parent seems to be medication-sensitive. If you identify depression and the doctor is not willing to entertain the possibility, be an outspoken advocate or find another doctor. Too many doctors view the elderly as "throw-away people." That sounds harsh, but it happens all too often.

Untreated depression in an older person can manifest as delusions and hallucinations. Some physicians will prescribe Haldol or some similar antipsychotic, when the actual drug of choice is an antidepressant. I have firsthand experience with this mistake.

My mother had a heart attack in 1995. Prior to that day she was experiencing some mild memory and vision loss, but was functioning alone during the day, handling the tasks of daily living without incident. She came out of the hospital with delusional dementia and remained that way for months. She was moved to an assisted living facility for her safety and my father's sanity. By chance, I heard of Dr. Jackson and her work in geriatric psychiatry.

Dr. Jackson did a complete work-up on Mom and determined that she had been suffering from untreated depression for years. She slowly took Mom off the antipsychotic, starting her on Prozac in the slow manner described above. Within four weeks Mom was a different woman. By twelve weeks she was vastly improved. Dr. Jackson explained that

untreated depression can manifest as delusions and hallucinations. The dementia cleared up somewhat, but did not
disappear, as it was due to oxygen loss during her heart
attack. With the long-overdue introduction of antidepressants, she functioned at a much-improved level.

Hers is not a story with a happy ending. The last
four months of my mother's life were a nightmare. She
screamed whenever any personal care was administered. No
one knew what was wrong. The staff could not find any
evidence of an injury that could account for her screaming. She was unable to verbalize what was happening to
her. Finally, the director of nursing told us she would
have to leave because she was too disruptive to the other
patients on the unit. She was transferred to a psychiatric
hospital for evaluation. They gave her enough medication
to calm her and transferred her to a nursing home, where
she refused to eat or drink. Because she had an Advance
Directive, she was not hydrated or fed through tubes or
IVs. She died in four days. After her death, when I went
back to the Alzheimer's unit to gather her things, I learned
she had been taken off her antidepressants. The hallucinations had come back as soon as the antidepressants were
out of her system. Her doctor, who had so carefully monitored her medications, had moved to New Jersey. It never
occurred to me that another doctor would arbitrarily alter
my mother's course of medication. She screamed for four
months and died in terror. It will take a lot of forgiveness
for me to let go of that one.

It is not unusual for the caregiver to need antidepressant medication. An antidepressant can be used for situational depression. It can be taken for six months to a year, then slowly withdrawn from the system. Usually the "green beans" are restored and the medication is no longer needed. If the depression reoccurs several times, long-term use of antidepressants may be advised.

Depression can often be a cause of memory loss in the elderly. A good antidepressant can improve their outlook on life and may drastically improve their memory. It is so exciting to see someone who has been depressed at a low level for many years "wake up" and start smiling. Anything to do with the brain may be resisted by your parent. They are not "crazy," they don't need "brain drugs." A good way to get past this mind-set is to describe depression as a severe form of stress. I know from my own experience that when I am under severe stress I have memory problems. We all do. It is God's way of protecting us from emotional overload. If a person is living under the gray cloud of depression, seeing no reason to get dressed in the morning, you can bet they are severely stressed.

You have nothing to lose and everything to gain by trying antidepressants for your parents or even yourself. The nice thing about antidepressants is that they work only if they are needed. If depression is not the problem, the drug will have no effect other than improved sleep. I repeat, depression is epidemic in the elderly. To leave a disease untreated that is so simple to treat is cruel and unbelievably stupid.

22

DEMENTIA:
WHO IS THE VICTIM?

As the daughter of a dementia victim, I could write tomes about my experience. Others have done the writing; I will share with you what I did not do soon enough and urge you not to make the same mistakes.

1. As soon as you see signs of dementia in your parent, call the Alzheimer's Association in your community or contact the national association. The address and phone numbers can be found in Part Five of this handbook. Alzheimer's disease is just one of fifty known causes of dementia, but it seems to be the catch phrase that covers all dementia. The association has books, videos, audio tapes, speaker schedules, classes and support groups for caregivers, and on and on. The more you understand about dementia, the better prepared you will be to give the best possible support to your parent, while remaining sane yourself.

2. Don't try to reason with a mind that can't reason. I tried
   to make my mother see how unreasonable her delusions
   were, and it only served to upset me. One day at her
   psychiatrist's office, I exploded at the social worker for
   agreeing with my mother's story about sleeping in a
   truck overnight and having all her clothes stolen. She
   took me aside and strongly suggested I get some help
   in understanding the disease. Until that day I had been
   in complete denial. Reason and logic do not have any
   impact on this disease. I had a terrible time understanding that basic fact. It seemed wrong to agree with delusions, but that is what we have to do.

3. Get involved in an Alzheimer's caregiver support group.
   Hospitals, churches, and the YWCA sponsor these
   groups in our local area—perhaps they do in yours, too.
   See Part Five of this book for the 800 number for the
   Alzheimer's Association. Meet others who are experiencing the same caregiving challenges. Get phone numbers
   of group members and keep "a sanity line" connected
   between you.

The national Alzheimer's Association has an application
for a Safe Return bracelet. At no cost, they will imprint
and send you an ID bracelet with your parent's name on
the top. On the back is an identification number for your
parent and the 800 number for the Safe Return program.
The bracelet is attractive, but impossible to open with one
hand, so your parent cannot remove it. Should your par-

ent become lost, the person who finds them calls the 800 number on the bracelet, and is put in touch with you so they can be safely returned home.

The National Caregiving Foundation, a division of the Alzheimer's Association, has a wonderful guide for the family caregivers, consisting of 114 pages of information plus cassette tapes. It provides information on the disease itself and training on how to respond to behaviors that puzzle and confound the family caregiver. It is free; all one must do is pick up the phone and call (800) 930-1357.

Home Instead Senior Care, nationally, has developed an excellent Alzheimer's Caregiver Training Program. There is a course of study, closed-book testing, and certification for the carefully selected caregivers who participate in the program. The company is gearing up to meet the growing needs of those who suffer from early-stage memory loss. A well-trained caregiver will not burn out when dealing with this very difficult disease. Before the training program, I was reluctant to take a memory-loss client. Now, with the soothing presence of caregivers who know just what to do in each situation, we are making a significant difference in quality of life for client and family.

~~~~~

The family who provides in-home care for a demented elderly person does the most difficult caregiving job any of us can ever imagine.

Jerry's story illustrates most of the issues. Jerry was

driven to an Alzheimer's support group as a last grasp on his sanity and his marriage. He and his wife, Leone, had been providing in-home care for his mother for nine years. His mother's illness had rapidly progressed in the past three years. Her confusion was such that she could not be left alone for a minute. Her personality had nearly disappeared. When she spoke, it was in a language only she could understand. She was incontinent and needed to be fed.

Nine years earlier, Jerry's mother had been charming, but confused enough to have difficulty with the tasks of daily living. The idea of in-home care did not seem daunting then. Jerry and Leone happily opened their home to her. They were now confronted with care that had long since stopped being a pleasure. They were caught in the trap so many families of dementia patients seem to fall into: they could not go on, but they could not let go.

Jerry and Leone were urged to consider a highly regarded dementia unit as a day-care resource. They took Mother there three days a week as a respite for themselves. To their surprise, she loved it. She absorbed the activity like a sponge takes up water. It was difficult for them to get her to leave at the end of the day.

Jerry and Leone finally saw that their sacrifice, as loving as it was, had kept Jerry's mother from being in a setting where she could "feel something." Mother had been as bored as Jerry and his wife had been exhausted. When they took into consideration her Social Security benefits and the money Jerry had wisely invested for her when her house was sold, Mother could afford to move into the Alzheimer's unit as a full-time resident.

This story is a perfect example of *"You are the jailer and you have the key."* For nine years Jerry had power of attorney for his mother. He was a signer on her checking and money market accounts. He let his guilt at "putting her in a home" keep him from investigating the existing resources. He had a mental picture of locked rooms and dark halls. On the contrary, Alzheimer's units are designed and operated with the goal of gentle stimulation for a diminishing mind. Go visit a unit. Observe the soft colors that are used. Many are designed in a circle so the residents never get lost. Soft music is used to soothe, and television is rarely turned on because of the rapidly changing screen images and the jarringly loud commercial messages.

From birth to adulthood, normal people follow a predictable pattern of development. At the onset of dementia, developmental achievements begin to disappear in reverse order. I have an Alzheimer's client who can no longer perceive danger. Our caregiver reported that the client was using sharp kitchen knives, and her husband was downplaying their risk. "She's used these knives for years, she's OK." I met with the spouse, described the reverse development aspect of his wife's disease, and asked him: if his five-year-old great-grandchild came to visit, would he put the knives out of reach and out of sight? Of course he would. I told him that his wife tried to catch a knife by the blade as it slipped through her fingers. Fortunately she was not cut because the knife handle hit the kitchen counter before her grip stopped its fall. Her perception of danger is at the level of a small child. She needs to be protected from sharp objects.

When memory loss progresses to the point where the client is no longer safe at home, the relationship of trust that we have built with the family allows us to help them make the difficult decision to move their parent to a secure facility where they can receive 24-hour care. Most clients make a speedy adjustment to being cared for in an environment that is designed for memory loss.

For the spouses who cannot let go of a loved one, all too often the caregiving spouse collapses from a stress-related illness. I have heard hundreds of spouses say they waited too long. The impaired spouse does better in a unit than they ever did at home. There is a chilling statistic in the *Journal of the American Medical Association,* December 15, 1999: A full-time caregiver has a 63 percent higher death rate than someone the same age, not involved in caregiving. If a parent or adult child caregiver insists upon dealing alone with dementia, go to the Web at www.jama.ama-assn.org and print the article, "Caregiving as a risk factor for mortality." That may be all you need to do to get their attention.

If you are caring for a dementia patient of any age, do so with the greatest possible help. If your father is providing in-home care for your mother or vice versa, encourage them to go to the Alzheimer's support groups. Help them to follow, step by step, the path described above with Jerry and Leoné. When one spouse cares for another, the caregiver is very likely to die first.

It helped me when I understood that at a certain point, I was the victim of the disease, not my mother. She was unable to sustain a thought long enough to be unhappy. Where did my mother go? I hope someone discovers the answer to that pretty soon.

23

WHAT IF ONE OF YOUR PARENTS TRULY IS A HORRIBLE PERSON?

I was in a women's group in San Francisco in the early eighties. It was the holiday season. Many of the members expressed their apprehension about going home for Christmas. I will never forget the therapist saying, "Hold it! There are four billion people on the face of the earth. That means there are four billion minus two that can fill your needs. Why do you continue behaving like a moth beating itself against a flame, expecting to enjoy the warmth but in fact getting killed? If you know it's going to be painful for you to be with your family, don't go. If you go, have realistic expectations. Don't set yourself up to believe that things are going to be different this time."

You know if the aging parent who needs your help is an emotionally or physically dangerous person. If your gut instinct is to stay away, then stay away. If you think you can help without being emotionally destroyed, help. There are ways to satisfy your personal need to do the right thing and at the same time take care of yourself, but it is a very fine line to walk and one you need to walk with great caution.

A parent who was mentally or physically abusive when you were a child is likely to be an abusive geriatric. If you hear yourself saying, "I know she is horrible, but she is my mother and she might need me," run for a therapist! Ultimately, only you know what you can do and what you must do. Sadly, all too often guilt overrules logic and judgment. Some damaged relationships cannot be mended. To try is to risk further damage.

A skill for coping with this dilemma can be to step back and ask, "What advice would I give a stranger?" Imagine that the stranger is someone you met on a cross-country train trip. Over several days of sitting together and sharing meals, the stranger lays out a history that sounds just like yours. If you gave her advice and suggestions, knowing you would never see her again, what would you tell her? Listen to your own advice. Can you heed it?

Trust your instincts. It may be that you can best help from a distance by sending a monthly check to contribute to caregiving expenses. Or, use your time and energy to research which social services are available to help your parent. The Yellow Pages for most communities in the United States are available on the Internet. They commonly have Senior Services grouped together on an easy-to-access list. A hospice social worker or a discharge planner at a local hospital are both wonderful resources. If you need to keep some distance, this is a positive way to do it. Your parent gets help, but you stay safe.

Kate, a nurse, tells a story about a man who was dying
in an intensive care unit. Though he had three children
and many grandchildren in the area, he was dying alone.
At the nurses' station there was a lot of talk about how sad
it was that Mr. Jones was all alone: "What kind of family
would leave a man to die alone?" Kate pointed out to her
colleagues that Mr. Jones may be a horrible person. He
could have abused his children. He could have driven their
mother to suicide. It is possible that to die alone is the
natural consequence of living with no regard for the needs
and feelings of others. Tough, yes. True, yes.

If we inflict unkindness and pain, it eventually comes
back to us in that form. Mr. Jones in the ICU would have
had his family gathered about him if he had enfolded them
in love and kindness. They could not respond to his illness
in any other way.

Like all healthy babies, Mr. Jones's children were born
with shiny eyes, laughter, and hope. We all know how
those happy babies grew into distant and self-protective
adults. We should be grateful that they were wise enough
to remain distant and self-protective. I am seriously concerned about adults who stay close to hateful people just
because they are family.

⌒

Jill's story describes the "mother from hell." Jill's mom
had bouts of serious depression throughout her life, taking

medication only as a last alternative to suicide. Jill and her brother, Michael, had been raised in an emotional time-bomb environment.

Michael had an inner strength that allowed him to survive their childhood more successfully than did Jill. He moved far away from the family just as soon as he was old enough to make it on his own. As often happens, the most damaged child stayed nearby. This mother-daughter relationship would sadden even the most jaded. As Mom grew older, her bouts of depression occurred more frequently. She would go for months without bathing, changing her clothes, or washing her hair. She suffered from malnutrition even though Jill saw to it that there was plenty of food in the house. As hard as she tried to help her mother, Jill's only reward was continued verbal abuse.

All her life, Jill had been the scapegoat. Jill was told she was responsible for all her mother's problems, responsible for everything that was wrong. She had heard it so long, she believed it. Through therapy, Jill began to understand that *anyone who was in the same room with her mother was going to be responsible for everything that was wrong.* Slowly, with determination, Jill separated herself from her mother physically and emotionally.

To make the final separation, Jill called upon Adult Protective Services to supervise Mom's medication and provide the services needed to assure her well-being. This was not an easy task. Jill was assertive and forceful in establishing that her mother was a danger to herself and thus legally fell under the umbrella of the protection of

Social Services. Mom was committed to a state psychiatric facility where her depression was treated. She was under care long enough for the antidepressants to take effect.

Jill consulted her brother before she gained the help of Adult Protective Services. Michael would show an interest in Mom's welfare if she would actually be getting some structured, professional help. Michael was the favored child, and his brief reappearance on the scene gave Mom a willingness to assemble some sort of life.

Jill has stayed completely away from her mother. She always keeps a kernel of hope that one day they can have some semblance of a healthy relationship. There is a partial happy ending to her story. Jill and Michael have developed a sibling relationship for the first time in their lives.

Jill's story illustrates that boundaries and sibling teamwork create results in the even the most tragic of circumstances. Working together, the brother and sister were able to facilitate a positive change in their mother's life while protecting themselves from continued emotional damage. Jill has learned to protect herself from all emotionally damaging relationships. Abused children can become abused or abusing adults. Jill had a series of relationships with men, which she can now look back on and say, "Of course they were jerks. I was an emotional sponge for their anger and rage. They saw me coming."

Jill's experience is a good example of the Chinese character for crisis, which is danger and opportunity intertwined. Through the resolution of the emotionally dangerous relationship with her mother, she was blessed with the opportunity to live a life she could never have imagined.

There is a spiritual phrase, "Namaste," which means, "The light in me recognizes the light in you." Every human being comes into this world with the "light" of love, kindness, and goodness available to him. No one is born with a character disorder. Even if there is a genetic predisposition toward mental illness, it is our life experiences that mold who each person becomes. We want to believe that at the end of a life, the light may again return, however briefly. Your desire to see this light may call you to the aid of a parent whom you might otherwise avoid. There are no hard and fast rules here. Be cautious. Listen to your instincts.

How many times have we said to ourselves, "I knew I this was going to happen," or, if we sidestepped a disaster, "I am so glad I followed my instincts." Remember that wise saying, "When I am doing what is right for me, I am doing what is right for everyone else in my life." This may sound self-serving, but it turns out to be true. Think about a major intersection in the road of your life. It takes courage to do what you know is right for you, especially if it is in opposition to what others think you should do. Looking back, you see how none of the good things that have happened to you would have happened had you not taken that road. The "coulda, shoulda, woulda's" are the way we describe taking the wrong road, *knowing* we should do one thing, but *doing* something else anyway. Trust that "knowing" inside of you; it seldom leads you down the wrong road.

The emotionally damaged adult child who brings this damage to a support group can drive away group members who are dealing with the normal issues of aging parent relationships. The group may be flowing along, everyone enriching each other with their problem-solving abilities, and in walks a new person who overwhelms the meeting with insoluble problems, while being unwilling to listen to any guidance. If this person continues to attend the group, it may be very difficult to keep the healthy members coming back. The damaged adult child who is stuck in the problem and unwilling to entertain any solution needs one-on-one professional help. If you are in a group like this, urge the facilitator to refer the damaged member to therapy. Otherwise, the group may dissolve.

If you are in a relationship with a parent who is dangerous to you emotionally or physically, find a therapist. Take care to choose one who is knowledgeable in the area of adult children of aging parents. A good marriage counselor does not necessarily make a good therapist for these issues. Do *not* let your fingers do the walking through the Yellow Pages. Call a geriatric care manager or the local Alzheimer's Association for referrals. Their numbers are listed in Part Five. Lack of money will not keep you from help. Every community has free or sliding-fee scale therapists who are very capable.

Holding resentment is like drinking poison and waiting for the other person to die!

PART FIVE

*Take Care of Yourself or
Sugar May Not Be the Answer!*

24

WHEN YOU COME TO
THE END OF YOUR ROPE

I find that my rope has different lengths. At times, I know my blood pressure is higher than it should be. When my parents were both in crisis, there were days when I was convinced that if I had one more problem to solve, if the phone rang one more time, or if one more thing was asked of me, I would get on a plane going anywhere and never return.

I learned that when i left my sweet, little mother in a locked facility surrounded by people who were as out of touch with the world as she was, it was sometimes more than I thought I could stand. If I were a drinker, I would have headed straight for a bar. I was more likely to head for Baskin Robbins. Neither of those coping skills is healthy. I can now identify the sugar craving as a stress-related insulin drop. I got better at reminding myself to carry a baggie of fruit in the car when I went on those excruciatingly difficult visits. Negative feelings are part

of life. Overload happens. The willingness to follow negative feelings toward emotional understanding is a healthy
response to stress.

The most common stress reactions are impatience and
anger. I learned many years ago that I am rarely angry
about what I think I am angry about. My irritation is
more often unidentified fear expressing as 'crooked anger.'
Crooked anger is when your boss comes out of a meeting where he has been outmaneuvered by his number-one
rival...and calls you incompetent when you ask him for
clarification on a project you're completing...so when you
leave the office, you criticize the security guard because his
uniform is soiled...and the guard is horrible to the clerk at
Safeway who has had too many nasty people come through
her check stand...then the clerk yells at her children to
pick up the mess in the living room, before she even says
hello...and her son kicks the dog. The final recipient of
your boss's fear and anger is the dog!

When you feel anger, identify the cause of those feelings *before* you snap at the next person you see. If the boss
in the endless sentence above had taken a moment to
identify his rudeness—as fear that his rival had just ended
his chances at becoming division manager—he would not
have been any happier, but he would have known it was
not your fault. Without crooked anger, your boss could
have greeted your question with, 'At this moment, if I had
a sledgehammer I would throw it through that plate glass
window! Give me half an hour will you?'

Overload happens when the anger layers become so

deep, we can barely cope. If we can identify each layer as it happens, even if we can't do anything about it, that layer can be set aside and the pile will not grow so deep that 'the dog gets kicked.'

When I ask myself, *What are you afraid of?* I can cut right to the root of the problem. You will never hear me say that it is easy to take a break in the middle of anger to ask myself that question, but when I do, I can save myself from an entire day of crooked anger. My husband has a wonderful soft style of reminding me to look under the anger. He is a very brave man.

⁓

Frustration is a common source of caregiver stress. Frustration usually arises from feelings of helplessness or incompetence. The overload that comes from frustration builds in the same layering manner as anger. Learning to isolate the offending incident or problem is the best stress management tool I know. The identifying phrases for frustration layers are: 'I can't do this; I don't know how; it's too much for me; *Why isn't this working?*' When these kinds of questions run through your mind, are you feeling helpless or incompetent? If so, what is the issue? You may not be able to change the situation, but knowing where the feelings are coming from can let the air out of the balloon.

I hire and place caregivers for a living. My overload can sometimes be seven caregivers deep. Client problems, caregiver problems, staffing problems can all hit at one time.

When this happens I must put away the folders, files, and notebooks that have piled up on my desk as each problem has been handed to me. When I clear the desk and work on one solution at a time, I have handled the overload. I am very visual. The 'pile of papers' that represent the problems creates the feeling of overload—not the problems themselves. The problems don't go away when I put the paper away. The mind clutter goes away so I can deal with one thing at a time. I can keep seven balls bouncing in the air at one time, but I can really only do one thing at a time.

Analyze your style. How do you manage overload? If you don't have a clue, look at the overload you are in at this moment. Visualize the 'stuff' whatever it is, as a pile of rocks. Your job is to remove the gravel, then the larger rocks, until you uncover the boulder that supports them all.

As an example, let's say the 'stuff' is moving your mother to a retirement community. She has lived in the same house for forty years. You have measured her apartment walls, looked at the cupboards and closets, and now it's downsizing time. The 'gravel' is the accumulated storage in the basement and attic that hasn't been touched in years. The 'rocks' are the contents of the closet, bathroom, and kitchen. The 'boulders' are the items your mother is so attached to that she will not be who she is if they don't move with her.

The gravel and the rocks are relatively easy to deal with; it is deciding which boulders to move that creates the core of the stress. When you look at the whole project, it is overwhelming. But, in fact, only about a dozen boulders and ten or fifteen boxes of rocks make up the real problem.

My friend Patricia saved my sanity when I was moving from Maui to Portland. I couldn't even articulate how overwhelmed I was. Patricia and I were driving from Kehei to Lahaina when she took out a notebook so we could list the things I had to do. For each item, she asked me to estimate how long it would take to accomplish. When we got through the list, it amounted to fifteen hours of actual time. I had two weeks to do fifteen hours of tasks. Instantly, my stress level dropped, and we went to the beach!

When something huge is looming before you, try the gravel, rocks, and boulders or the time-estimate overload management tools. They have never failed me.

Develop coping tools that work for you. My favorite stress escape is reading. The higher the stress, the more I read. I like 'airplane books.' A well-written mystery or John Grisham novel can entertain me for hours. Books on tape are wonderful for occupying my thoughts while driving or doing household tasks. *It is important for my mind to go someplace where worry cannot invade.* The public library has an endless supply of novels and tapes. When I read for stress relief, I don't read or listen to anything educational. This is escape, pure and simple.

Creating music is another coping tool that regenerates

my spirit. Singing can increase my energy level faster than a nap. I learned the music coping skill when my children were school age. I used to tell them, 'Short of death or dismemberment, do not disturb me while I practice the guitar.' Learning to play a guitar required total concentration. The four of them would actually leave me alone for about forty-five minutes, which was just long enough for me to give the guitar lesson total attention and regain my sanity before their father got home from work.

The 'death or dismemberment' line seemed to be funny enough, yet strong enough, for them to take seriously. Over the years, 'death or dismemberment' became a lexicon of the family. If I used those words, I could go into my bedroom, shut the door, and lie down for a few minutes. There are magic words for you too. Find them. You have to be able to express your needs in a way that people can hear your words, and take you seriously.

We all know that diet and exercise are important. It is never too late to lose twenty pounds, exercise regularly, eat a balanced diet...all the things that are good for us and that are seemingly the last things we ever want to do. Why is that? If anyone comes up with an answer to that dilemma, I want to know about it.

Walking can place me in a revitalized frame of mind in a very short time. I love to walk through my neighborhood, remodeling the exterior of homes that could use a face-lift. I add shutters, tear out shrubs, replace old windows with vinyl...all inside my head.

The families I work with report that even a short walk

around the block will bring back a semblance of emotional balance when the pressures of caregiving have them at the end of their ropes. Walking and breathing, letting your mind go somewhere other than back to the immediate problem is, in fact, a lifesaver. Stress-related illness is likely to kill a family caregiver before or shortly after the person being cared for. This is especially true when caring for someone afflicted with dementia. Finding your route to managing stress is vital.

My first instinct when my parent's needs began to demand more of my time was to cancel all nonessential activities. I quickly learned this was not the way to live my life. It was evident that dropping all the people and activities I enjoyed was a sure downward spiral into depression. The 'outside world' keeps me sane—tired, but sane. The good news about being tired is, sleep comes easily.

It may have been a long time since you gave serious thought to what you like to do. Life has a way of scheduling us into a routine that can take the life out of living. Finish these sentences:

I absolutely love to _____

_____.

It is has been so long since I _____

_____.

If I had time, I would _____

_____.

Fill in the blanks, and then start making time for *you* in your life. It is like setting a boundary. You start with small steps and pretty soon, you have altered your life pattern.

Each of us has our own path to pleasure and relaxation. I have a friend who went horseback riding in Montana for two weeks. That is the last thing I would ever do, but she came back refreshed and renewed. My husband read *Chaos Theory* on the deck of the QE 2. Why would anybody choose to do that?

25

WE ARE ALL DOING
EXACTLY WHAT WE
WANT TO DO

A number of years ago I attended a sales training seminar. I was the only woman in the room, surrounded by a lot of 'three-piece suits.' At the end of the afternoon, the final speaker was a psychologist whose message nearly cleared the room. He opened with: 'We are all doing exactly what we want to do.' I was sitting in the third row, and I watched the color rise on the necks of the men in front of me. Their response was an angry, 'You don't understand, I have responsibilities and obligations. I am not doing what I want to do, I am doing what I have to do.' They nearly tarred and feathered the speaker.

He listened patiently and said, 'Every one of you are physically and financially capable of walking out of this room, going to the airport, and taking the first flight to Hawaii, and, if you have a passport, the first flight to the gold coast of Australia. You can do that. You make choices in your life moment by moment. You are the jailer and you have the key. I am not suggesting that you dump your family, quit your job, and get on a plane. I am asking you to seriously consider that *you could do that if you wanted to.* If you understand that concept, you will be much more accepting of what you choose moment by moment. You have absolute freedom. You must be willing to accept the consequences that come with that freedom, but you do have absolute freedom.'

When I find myself feeling trapped, I think of that psychologist. I don't even remember his name, but he changed my attitude forever. I do have choices. I have taken all sorts of risks and gone down roads less traveled. There have been consequences, but my life is full of life.

We hear a lot about stress and its negative effects. Stress in itself is not negative. Our *response* to stress is what makes it problematic. In his book, *The Survivor Personality.* Al Siebert, Ph.D., discusses the concept of 'illness-susceptible versus illness-resistant' personalities. He compares stress to the human body's allergic reaction to certain foods or drugs. If I were allergic to dairy products, my cells would react to those substances as if they were poison. The cells would go into a catatoxic reaction to destroy the poison. I am not allergic to dairy products, so my cells interpret milk as being not harmful. The cells have a syntoxic reaction. The cells put up with the milk, even gain nourishment from it.

Some people have allergic minds. They feel alarmed and distressed about many ordinary events. Others have emotional immunities to those circumstances. They convert the events into something that nourishes them.

The good news is: it is easier to alter our thinking than to alter our cellular reactions. At the same time, our thinking can alter our cells, as witnessed by those who have visualized actual healing experiences. But first we have to get control of our thinking. I am convinced that life is 10 percent what happens, and 90 percent how we react to it. We can change the power of any situation by changing how we view it.

There is a Taoist story about a man of great wisdom whose horse ran away across the border into a neighboring country. When the villagers came to console him, he responded, 'What makes you think this isn't a blessing?' The next spring, his horse returned, bringing four other horses with it. When the villagers came to congratulate the man on his good fortune, he said, 'What makes you so sure this is not a disaster?' The man had a son who loved to ride the horses, and one day he was crippled in a riding accident. When the villagers tried to console the man on the misfortune of his only son, he replied, 'What makes you think this isn't a blessing?' A year later, an enemy invaded the man's country, and every able-bodied young man went into battle. Nine of ten warriors were killed. Only because of the earlier accident had both father and son survived to take care of each other. Blessings turn into disasters, and disasters become blessings—the changes go on forever. The mystery cannot be explained.

I have a strong survivor personality. Part of it was the gift of birth, but most of it was learning how to think differently. When I was thirty-six years old I had a 'broken coper.' I couldn't cope with spilled milk on the kitchen floor. Today, I am confident I can cope with anything.

Learning how to think differently requires effort. It requires reading, support or therapy groups, and individual therapy when the issues are clinical. It requires a spiritual shift. Everything you need to make you resilient enough to handle anything is within your reach. Look for the settings in which you can grow. If I can do it, you can do it. That is the secret of the survivor: 'Anything one person has done, I can do.' If you believe that, nothing can ever stand in your way.

Many of my friends and family thought I was crazy to buy a franchise for Home Instead Senior Care at sixty years of age. I was practically old enough to be my own client! But it was the perfect thing for me to do. I was slowly leaking life-force. That is the only way I can describe it. I was happy with my life, my marriage, my children, my friends, my volunteer activities—but I was not challenged. I was not using all the skills and talent God had given me. I needed a life purpose that was larger than my life. I found it.

I knew my field was going to be aging or adult children of the aging, because I was personally involved in both areas. My working background was in human services, so my resume would reinforce the direction I was taking. I knew I was on the right train—but was it on the right track? Where to go from there? My husband and I were going to a Bob Proctor Seminar, and we'd been asked to arrive with an idea to work on. (*Chicken Soup for the Soul* is a result of the Proctor Seminar.) Four weeks before the seminar, the universe dropped Home Instead Senior Care in my lap. I had found my direction.

I work for the forgotten seniors. I call my clients 'forgotten' because they are not *really* ill, nor *overly* frail, or *terribly* memory impaired, but they are beginning to need help. Inside their heads is a recurring thought: 'This is really getting hard to do, but if I ask for help that means I really need help, and if I need the help that means I am getting old...oh no, not me.' Those 'almost-elderly' seniors are my clients. In ten years, Home Instead Senior Care has become the largest nonmedical home-care provider in the world. As of this printing, we have 314 franchises in the United States, Japan, Canada, and Portugal. Why is this happening at such a remarkable growth rate? Because people want to age in place.

Older people want to stay home with their familiar lives and routines. The 'almost elderly' need help to accomplish this goal. They don't need a lot of attention, just enough to keep things running smoothly. The average client of Home Instead Senior Care receives twelve hours of caregiving weekly. That is enough time to get help with the groceries, laundry, errands, light housekeeping, getting to doctor appointments, the hairdresser, etc. We do not exclude clients who need more than twelve hours of help a week. I have several clients whom my caregivers see daily. Our line in the sand is *nonmedical care.* When nursing services are needed, I step aside and the nurses take over.

Someone asked me, 'What is your elevator speech?' I describe us as a 'rent-a-sibling' service. We do the tasks your sister would do for your parents. If my caregiver walks in the house and there are dishes in the sink, she does them. If she opens the refrigerator and something has turned into a chemistry experiment, she throws it away. If her client has a doctor appointment, she goes with him. If her client is returning home after being in a rehab center, she stays overnight for a few nights.

The clients I work with are at this almost-elderly stage. When your parents reach this stage, you may feel like you are walking on eggshells. You're trying to be careful not to hover over them, but at the same time, you don't want to overlook their increasing needs. Your mother may be perfectly capable of finding her way around her kitchen with her eyes closed, but she may need help going to the grocery store. Dad is perfectly capable of driving to the beach, but completely intimidated by his doctor. It is important to ask them frequently if there is anything that they need.

Ask them if you are doing too much or not enough. Use those words. Reassure them that you do not see them as incapable, you just know that cleaning out the gutters on the roof may be a bit of a stretch! Communicate regularly. Health problems can come on rapidly, but you may not hear about them unless you ask. Keep your eyes and ears open. Be available, but don't hover. Suggest that they might enjoy having help once or twice a week. They may accept help from a stranger, but not from you. They don't want to 'be a burden' to you, but if they are paying for help, they can be a 'burden' if they want to. Your parents will remain independent much longer if they are supported in the tasks of daily living.

I am having a wonderful time with Home Instead Senior Care. My clients are glowing under the attention they receive. Families are feeling released from being supermen or wonderwomen, and our caregivers feel the pride of making a difference in everyone's life. I bound out of bed in the morning. I love what I do.

26

HELP IS OUT THERE!

Consider the woman who thinks she can work full time, keep her house clean, do the grocery shopping, cook the meals, do the laundry, take her seventeen-year-old to soccer practice, and while he is at practice, do the grocery shopping for her mother? On her day off, she watches her son play soccer, runs to her mother's to clean her house, does a couple loads of laundry, and cooks enough food to fill up the freezer for another week.

Wonderwoman will keep this up until a physical ailment or opportunistic accident puts her in bed for two weeks. Then, guess what she will do? She will start all over again. Are you cringing? I hope so. What makes us so blind? We don't seem to consider consequences to ourselves. We do what we think is right and get lost in all the busyness.

Instead, do your caregiving with love and commitment to your parents *and to yourself*. Only in recent years have the needs of the family caregiver been considered. The extent of stress-related illness in the caregiver has given rise to a network of support resources.

Medical research into stress has found it to be the cause of many illnesses, but studies also support a strong mind-body connection for wellness. By changing the way we think, we can begin to change the way we behave, thus saving our own lives and sanity. Try a support group. Nothing is more lifesaving than a room full of people who know how you feel, who will laugh and cry with you and be there for you with help and emotional support. This process brings 'Eskimos' into our lives; which leads me into one of my favorite stories.

Two men were seated in a bar in Alaska. One was a priest, the other an atheist. The priest asked the atheist why he didn't believe in God. The atheist answered that he gave God a final chance ten years ago. 'I was forty miles north of town in a blizzard. I got down on my knees and shouted, 'God, if there is a God, I am lost and I'm going to die...' The priest interrupted him, saying, 'Of course you believe in God, you're here aren't you?' The atheist shook his head and argued, 'No, it wasn't God. An Eskimo came along and showed me the way!'

Our lives are filled with 'Eskimos.' People come into our lives with answers if we can just be open to hearing them. Adult Children of Aging Parents and Alzheimer's support groups contain Eskimos. The group has healing power. We listen to the problems of another, search our brains for solutions for them, and in that process we find our own answers. *It is magic.* Do not walk this road alone. These groups can save your sanity.

Assisted living centers, Alzheimer's units, and retirement centers are good resources for finding family support groups. The social work department of your local hospital will have resource listings for your community and will be happy to help. They may be willing to start and facilitate a group, if requested. Large medical centers will have an entire department for caregiving, with patient and family support groups for everything from arthritis to alcoholism. Geriatric psychiatrists and psychologists usually have support groups within their practices, or can lead you to groups that meet in your community.

Social workers in hospice programs are a great resource. You can find Hospice in the Yellow Pages or through your local hospital. They will likely have group support, consistent with hospice's focus on taking care of the families of their patients.

The local YWCA and YMCA will have therapists on staff who may be persuaded to facilitate an ACAP group. It is the sort of work they do, so the idea should be well received. If they cannot provide a therapist, they may at least be able to provide space for the group to meet.

So care for yourself as well as your parents. There is a way to have it all: You don't have to do it all!

27

CONTACTS
AND RESOURCES

SUPPORT SERVICES

Alzheimer's Association
(800) 272-3900   www.alz.org
   This dedicated group of paid and volunteer staff provides books, videos, pamphlets, and scientific studies to help you understand why dementia happens, how it affects your parents, how it will affect you, and how you can help without going off the deep end yourself. They provide a meeting place and a facilitator for Alzheimer's support groups for family and patients. A newsletter keeps you informed about upcoming events as well as the newest research and medications. An application for the Safe Return bracelet (described in Part Four) can be obtained by calling their 800 number.

Children of Aging Parents (CAPS) National Information and Referral Line
(800) 227-7294   www.experts.com

CAPS is a nonprofit organization that provides information and emotional support to caregivers of older people. It is a national clearinghouse for information on resources for the elderly. CAPS will direct you to an adult children's support group in your area.

⌒

National Council on the Aging
(202) 479-1200   (800) 424-9046   www.ncoa.org
409 Third St., SW, Second Floor, Washington, DC 20024

National Council on the Aging is a clearing house for resources, statistics and research as well as a source for publications on specific issues of aging.

⌒

Home Instead Senior Care
(888) 484-5759   www.homeinstead.com

Home Instead Senior Care is accessible nationally. They provide nonmedical services such as companionship, meal preparation, light housekeeping, laundry, errands, and incidental transportation. The service is private pay. Caregivers are carefully screened, bonded, and insured.

⌒

National Association of Private Geriatric Care Managers
(520) 881-8008   www.caremanager.org

Geriatric care managers will assess your parent's condition; look at medications; make recommendations for change, if necessary; and refer you to individuals or companies that provide in-home care. They will also interface with a physician on your behalf. Call for a guide ($15.00) that lists CGMs by state.

Area Agency on Aging
(800) 677-1116   www.n4a.org

This nationwide Eldercare Locator is an information and referral source provided by the U.S. Administration on Aging and administered in cooperation with the National Association of State Units on Aging. There are resources for every zip code in the country. You can locate Alzheimer's hotlines, adult day care, respite services, nursing home ombudsman assistance, and legal services; or report consumer fraud or make in-home care complaints, and research many more topics.

American Academy of Home Care Physicians
(410) 676-7966   www.aahcp.org
Email is aahcp@mindspring.com

This established group of physicians who see their

patients *where they are* is growing by leaps and bounds. They are proactively getting ready to serve the needs of the burgeoning aging population. This is the new generation of Dr. Welbys.

⸻

National Caregiving Foundation (Division of the Alzheimer's Association)
(800) 930-1357 (Leave your name and address and the guide will arrive in 3-4 weeks)

This is an excellent training guide for any family member or private caregiver. It provides, at no cost, a 114-page, three-ring binder plus cassette tapes, which give excellent training in how to understand and manage this difficult disease. You may make a donation to the Foundation upon receipt of the guide, if you wish.

⸻

There are also Internet sites that offer endless links to services for elders and their children. You can find them at:

www.careguide.com (Careguide Eldercare Locator)
www.aarp.org/caregivers
www.caregivers.net
www.elderconnect.com
www.rivendell.org
www.americangeriatrics.org

FURTHER READING

Every book requires research. I came upon several wonderful books while writing this one, which I encourage you to read. Each of them is unique in content.

I will tell you the story that led me to one of the recommended books, *Your Best Is Good Enough*. In 1996 my husband and I were having lunch in the Sultan's Palace in Istanbul. A couple from New Jersey joined us and asked me, 'What do you do?' I answered that I was writing a handbook for adult children of aging parents. The wife asked if I had read Vivian Greenberg's book, *Your Best Is Good Enough*. I replied that I hadn't, but I would certainly find it when I got home.

I did, only to discover that Vivian Greenberg had written my book! I liked her book so well that I put mine into what I thought was permanent computer storage and ordered two dozen copies of *Your Best Is Good Enough* for a workshop I was organizing. After corresponding and talking with Vivian on the subject, she told me, 'Suzanne, I didn't write your book. Your book reflects you and your unique outlook.' Thankfully, I listened to her.

Your Best Is Good Enough (renamed by the publisher to) *Respecting Your Limits When Caring for Aging Parents* by Vivian Greenberg ($19.95, hardcover). To order, call Jossey-Bass Inc., Publishers, at (800) 956-7739.

Another Country by Mary Pipher, PhD. Available in major

bookstores. Mary (author of Reviving Ophelia) does a masterful job of describing the world of the elderly, the 'landscape of old age.'

Children of a Certain Age by Vivian Greenberg. Discusses the interaction between generations and how adult children and aging parents can relate to each other to heal old wounds. Available from Jossey-Bass Inc., (800) 956-7739.

A Long Goodbye and Beyond by Linda Combs, Ed.D. An in-depth treatment of the subject. Published by Book Partners, Inc. Call to order, (800) 895-7323.

What to Do When Mom Moves In by Betty Kuhn. This is an A to Z look at all the aspects of caring for a parent. Also available from Book Partners, Inc. Call to order, (800) 895-7323.

Coping With Your Difficult Older Parent: A Guide for Stressed Out Children by Grace Lebow, Barbara Kane, with Irwin Lebow. Published by Avon Books. Call to order (800) 238-0658

Circles of Care by Ann Cason is a loving book from inside the caregiving experience. Cason helps us understand how to focus on the strengths, not the weaknesses, of patients and their caregivers. Published by Shambhala Press, www.shambhala.com.

Caregiving: The Spiritual Journey of Love, Loss and Renewal by Beth McLeod, published by John Wiley and Sons. Nominated for a Pulitzer Prize, this book is both practical (with action steps at the end of each chapter) and spiritual.

The 36-Hour Day by Nancy Mace and Peter Rabins, published by Johns Hopkins University Press. This is the most well-known book for caregivers of dementia victims.

A great deal has been written since, but this book remains the groundbreaker.

28

DEATH:
THE FINAL CHAPTER

Being a caregiver moves us into introspection and the awareness of our needs and the needs of others. We develop all sorts of coping skills we might never have learned had our parents died when we were twenty-five. After being the catalysts who have brought us all these gifts, inevitably our parents die.

Elisabeth Kubler-Ross has brilliantly defined the stages of grief we all must pass through, taking us from denial to acceptance. I will suggest that there is one stage she has not defined. This stage happens to those of us who have been caregivers. That stage is relief.

The funeral is over, the relatives and friends have gone home, you are now able to make plans for tomorrow that will not include caregiving responsibilities. You don't need to run by Mom's to drop off the sweater you picked up at the cleaners. You don't have to try to reach her doctor. You don't have to go to the nursing home today.

If you were doing caregiving in your home, the change will be even more dramatic. You don't have to deal with adult undergarments today. You do not have to be awakened four times tonight. You don't have to answer the same question five times while remaining patient and kind.

Your life will now have a rhythm you can set. The relief is real, it is good, and it is reasonable to feel it. You can have positive and negative feelings at the same time. This has nothing to do with your not loving your parent, or wishing you could have done more (which is the guilt stage of grief). It just is. It is normal and natural to feel relief.

If you can afford it, go to a health spa for a week, get massages, a manicure, pedicure, and facial. If you love golf, go to your favorite resort and play five rounds of golf. Go to the beach and walk along the shore. Celebrate the completion of a job well done in whatever way suits your life. Don't get up and go to work as usual! Give yourself time to reflect on your capacity to love another person. Pat yourself on the back and relax for a while. Don't immediately go and clean out your parent's house to get it on the market for sale. Don't do anything that is project driven. Breathe, relax, and let the relief wash over you.

One last piece of practical advice: don't go to the estate sale at your parents' house. After the family has chosen their favorite mementos, the time comes when you must place the physical items of your parents' lifetimes into the hands of strangers. Hire a professional with good references to price and sell the items. If there are expensive items in your parents' home, such as antiques or original art, turn them over to reputable dealers or galleries who can appraise and sell them for you.

I have heard adult children describe watching strangers paw through their parent's treasured possessions. A dishtowel that was embroidered by Aunt Helen could have been a treasured item to your mom, but when a stranger tosses it aside because of a stain, you will feel the pain. Be very careful how you care for yourself during this time of early mourning.

———◦

Congratulations! You have read this entire handbook. You have laughed, cried, considered, disagreed, and learned a great deal in these pages. You have come to the banquet table, helping yourself to what you needed. Put this book away for a while. When you open it again, the information will seem to have changed because you will have changed. Later, when you are hungry, angry, lonely, or tired, you can return to refill your plate.

ABOUT THE AUTHOR

As owner of the West Portland and Beaverton, Oregon, franchises of Home Instead Senior Care, Suzanne Roberts works with adult children every day. Her caregiving staff provides nonmedical, in-home care for the elderly. She recognizes the stress and overwhelm in the children of her clients as feelings she experienced herself when caring for her aging parents.

When Suzanne discovered Home Instead Senior Care, she assessed her degree in Human Services and her career skills in medical staff recruiting, counseling, intervention, and employee assistance—and knew everything she had ever learned would be utilized as she pursued this new direction for her life. Today, Suzanne says, 'If I won the lottery, I would do exactly what I'm doing now—except I'd pay my caregivers more!'

In the four years between the date of publication and the third edition, Suzanne has kept a very busy schedule. She has been a featured guest for interview and talk formats on radio and television. Her appearances have ranged from a 2-1/2-minute spot on the noon news in Seattle to the half hour guest spot on a national radio talk show. Suzanne has spoken to audiences from Florida to Washington State. Her offerings range from a 45-minute keynote address to a half-day workshop. Suzanne facilitates the monthly Children of Aging Parents meeting for Legacy Hospitals in Portland. She has spoken to dozens of family and professional groups locally and nationally. She has even turned her information around for presentation to aging parents, as they deal with their children!!

TO CONTACT
SUZANNE ROBERTS

Mail

PO Box 1605
Portland, Oregon 97207

Fax

(503) 245-3909

E-mail

coping@suzanneroberts.net

Web site

www.suzanneroberts.net

To order
additional copies of
Coping in New Territory

Price
$13.95 USA
$16.95 Canada

Shipping
$3.50 for first copy
$2.00 each additional copy up to 5 copies

Discounts
Quantity discounts are available by request.
Contact the author by fax or e-mail.

Available at all bookstores or major bookstore web sites
or through the author's web site at
www.suzanneroberts.net.